HUSBANDRY AND MANAGEMENT PRACTICES IN FARROWING UNITS II

Lactation

Property of:

© 2015 Grupo Asís Biomedia S.L.
Plaza Antonio Beltrán Martínez, nº 1, planta 8 - letra I
(Centro empresarial El Trovador)
50002 Zaragoza - Spain

First edition: April 2015

Illustrator:
Jacob Gragera Artal

Translation:
Melissa Testa

ISBN: 978-84-16315-10-9
D.L.: Z 552-2015

Design and layout:
Servet editorial - Grupo Asís Biomedia S.L.
www.grupoasis.com
info@grupoasis.com

Warning:

Veterinary science is subject to constant evolutionary change. It is therefore the veterinary surgeon's inescapable responsibility, based on his/her professional experience, to determine and verify the dosage, method, period of administration and contraindications of the treatments applied to each patient.
Neither the publisher nor the author assume any liability for injury and/or damages to persons, animals or property arising from the use or misapplication of the data shown in this work.

HUSBANDRY AND MANAGEMENT PRACTICES IN FARROWING UNITS II

Lactation

Emilio Magallón Botaya (coordinator)
Alberto García Flores
Roberto Bautista Moreno
Boris Alonso Sánchez
José Ignacio Cano Latorre
Patricia Prieto Martínez
Pablo Magallón Verde

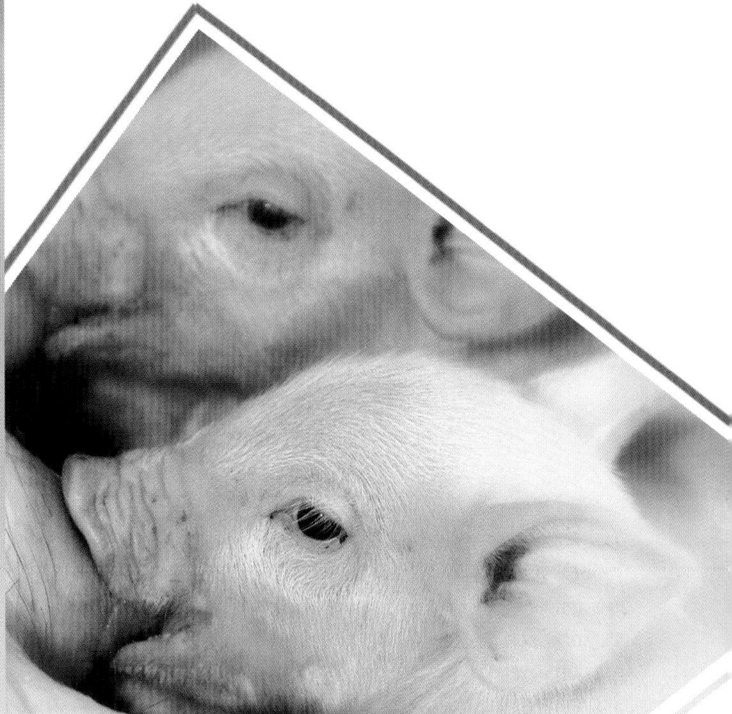

SERVET

To our parents, because their example of work, sacrifice and affection has served as a model to educate our children.

AUTHORS

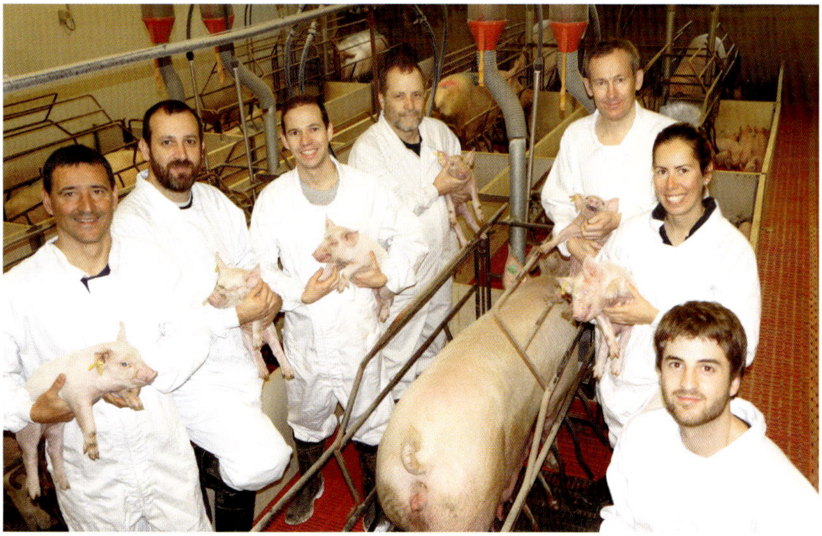

The authors of this book are a group of professionals of the swine industry, all of them qualified veterinary surgeons, who work for one of the main pig production companies in Spain.

In addition to their university degree in veterinary medicine, they have done several master's degrees and courses in animal health and production both in Spain and other countries. They have an in-depth knowledge of the different aspects of pig production, from farm facilities to environmental control, genetics, nutrition, health and management, as well as production costs and personnel management.

They have visited the main pig-producing countries worldwide to know the different production systems in situ.

Their technical knowledge and extensive practical experience –acquired through their daily work on farms in collaboration with farmers– is reflected in this book and will hopefully help readers manage modern farrowing units, especially during the lactation period, in the ever-changing and competitive sector of pig production.

PROLOGUE

It is an honour to write the foreword to this book, dedicated to the productive phase of lactation. I greatly enjoyed this book for two reasons: firstly, it reminded me of my early years as a farm veterinary surgeon, during which I worked in close relationship with the authors; and secondly, the quality of its contents is extraordinary and perfectly reflects the rigour of the authors' undeniable practical knowledge.

The topic addressed, lactation, has important implications both for the sow and her piglets, and will greatly influence the operation's subsequent productivity levels. For the sow, maximising her voluntary feed intake will be crucial to maximise her subsequent performance. Productive differences between the different countries partly result from an incapacity to achieve a standard and uniform environmental control throughout the whole year, with the negative impact of the summer season. This aspect influences the sow's voluntary feed intake negatively during lactation, which in turn has a negative impact on both her fertility and subsequent prolificacy. It also has an impact on piglets, whose weaning weight is closely related to their mother's milk production, which depends on her voluntary feed intake. Weaning weight will also influence the main performance parameters related to efficiency in the transition and fattening stages.

Given the impact of lactation on the performance and efficiency of sows and piglets during the transition and fattening stages, the practical advice contained in this book can be used as a base to achieve their optimisation.

To conclude, I would like to highlight the fantastic work carried out by all the authors, whose dedication and professionalism are reflected in every chapter of this book. In addition, I would also like to mention the participation of Emilio Magallón, the coordinator of this project, who has contributed to making this book see the light of day. I am convinced you will love it.

Luis Miguel Laborda Usan
Veterinary surgeon, specialist in Swine Genetics and Production

FOREWORD

After more than 20 years in the pig industry, we still work with the same enthusiasm we had when we started our professional career. This is due to the fact that pig production is constantly evolving, and has done so more particularly in the past few years thanks to genetic progress, new feeding protocols, health and biosecurity programmes, new farm facilities and equipment...

Moreover, thanks to the Internet boom and access to research studies through specialised journals, talks, papers, etc., a large amount of information is now available to us, but it is often of little use as it cannot be applied on our farms.

We live in an increasingly globalised world and must be very competitive if we want to stay in the business.

Changes take place so rapidly that we always feel like we are one step behind the best farms, with few possibilities to catch them up. To do so, it is necessary to be willing to introduce changes, to innovate (if we keep doing things in the same way, we will keep getting the same results). For this reason, and based on our experience, we would like to encourage you to do it.

This book is aimed mainly at swine farmers, to help them improve their farm's management strategies at so crucial a stage of production as lactation. It can also be useful to swine technicians, farrowing unit supervisors and workers, as another tool to standardise processes in farrowing rooms and optimise farm production.

For people like us who are more used to learning than to teaching, to reading than writing...., it has not been easy to summarise our own knowledge and that of others to write this book. We have used many graphs, pictures and tables to make it easier to read and understand, without leaving out the scientific grounds of the topics addressed. We hope to have achieved our objective.

Nacho Cano Latorre

ACKNOWLEDGEMENTS

To our families, for their patience, affection and priceless support, which have allowed us to get this book –the result of great dedication and commitment– off the ground.

To all the veterinary practitioners and professionals of the sector who have shared their knowledge and actively collaborated with us, especially our colleagues at Inga Food for their dedication, commitment, energy and in short, for being who they are.

To the professionals on swine operations with whom we work in close relationship and who help us increase our knowledge on a daily basis.

To Grupo Asís for their professionalism when guiding us in this new project.

To all those who have crossed our paths with a positive attitude and challenged us with new objectives, by showing us new ways of doing things, which has allowed us to rethink some essential concepts and progress in our knowledge.

TABLE OF CONTENTS

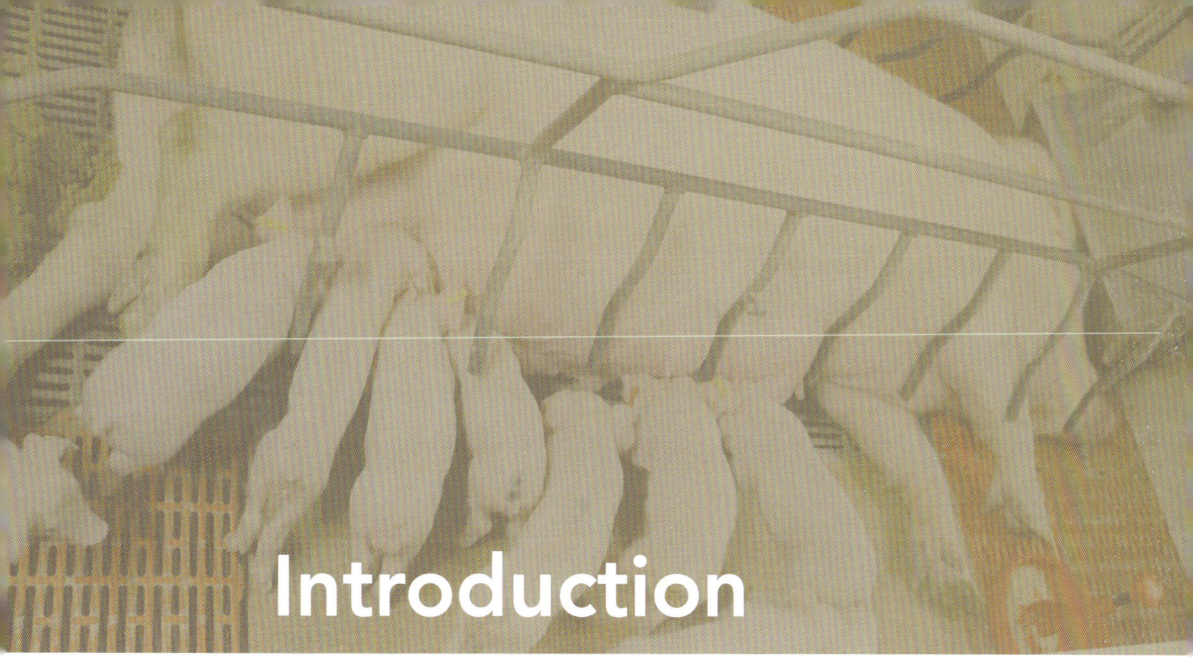

Introduction

Sow farms have been undergoing considerable changes over the past few years: increase in the average size of operations; new, more prolific genetic lines; health status improvements; better-qualified personnel; changes in feeding practices; improved facilities...

All these changes have increased sow farm productivity worldwide significantly.

The best operations produce more than 30 piglets per productive sow and year; some even exceed 33 piglets. In Denmark, some operations wean more than 38 piglets per productive sow and year.

These spectacular increases in productivity require new husbandry and management concepts in all areas of pig production, but particularly in farrowing houses. Sows farrow more but smaller piglets, and the new swine maternal lines are leaner, have a greater mammary development, produce more milk and need a good body condition to be able to nurse all their offspring. This results in longer and more productive lactation periods and requires changes in feeding programmes, facilities, sow and piglet management, personnel management...

This book starts with the technical and physiological aspects of lactation to then focus on environmental control in farrowing units, animal welfare, sow and piglet feeding and sow management during lactation, with a special focus on cross-fostering and weaning. It also addresses the main diseases in this period as well as personnel management, and ends with some conclusions and a list of references.

This book is pleasant and easy to read, but it is based on rigorous scientific research; numerous pictures, diagrams and summaries have been used to present the information given.

We, the authors of this book, are professionals of the sector who are very involved in the daily work on sow farms. We have therefore chosen to avoid overly technical terms and used an accessible and simple language.

This book is aimed at a very heterogeneous audience, from veterinary professionals to students, unit supervisors, farm workers specialised in farrowing unit management and, of course, all those livestock professionals who would like to know the state of the art in farrowing unit management on modern sow farms in a quick and straightforward manner.

Our approach for this book was chosen with all these people in mind, as we aimed to summarise the scientific grounds for husbandry and management practices in lactation –a crucial phase of a farm's global production process–, as well as the innovations achieved in this area in the past few years.

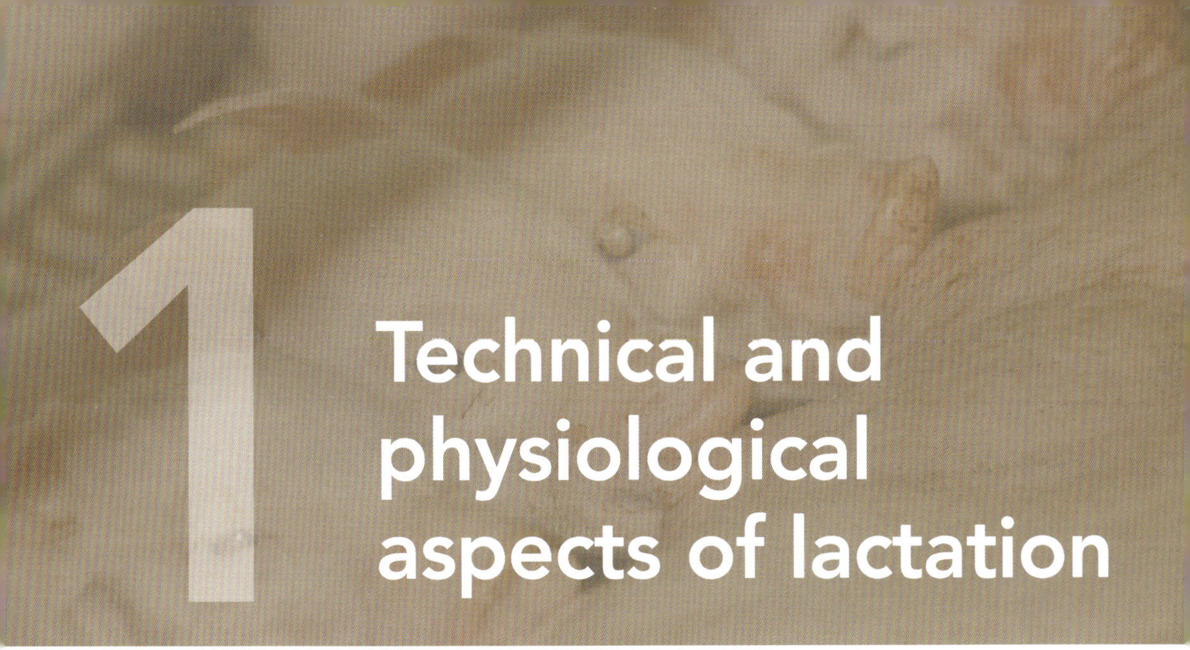

1 Technical and physiological aspects of lactation

Natural behaviour of the sow and piglet during lactation

Nursing

Immediately after the birth of her piglets, the sow already has colostrum available in her udders, since high oxytocin levels (hormone involved in milk ejection) are reached after farrowing. From the first day postpartum, colostrum secretion progressively ceases while milk secretion starts; milk is not available continually, which requires the piglets to massage and stimulate the mammary glands to induce milk ejection. At the beginning, nursing occurs every 40-60 minutes, although it decreases as the lactation period progresses.

Short after their birth, piglets compete with each other in order to establish their social hierarchy. As a result, the largest and more vigorous piglets suckle at the thoracic teats, which are the most productive. Once the hierarchy is established, piglets always suckle at the same teat. Piglets choose a teat from their second day of life; they seem to guide themselves through the smell of the saliva they leave on the teat.

> The largest and more vigorous piglets suckle from the most productive teats, as a result of the hierarchical order established by competition between the members of the litter.

Behaviour of the sow in the farrowing room

The behaviour of sows with their piglets has an influence on neonatal mortality rates, especially as regards the risk of crushing. The sows that remain in lateral recumbent position allow their piglets better access to their teats. Thus, the sows that move less and do not make sudden movements prevent many deaths by crushing from occurring (Fig. 1). Sows with inappropriate behaviour increase mortality rates.

There is a clear relationship between sows with a good behaviour (good mothers) and productivity.

How dangerous a sow's movements are depends on how careful she is when lying down, how suddenly she does so and where the piglets are at that moment. The danger a sow represents varies according to the environmental conditions and the time of the day.

Piglets in danger usually make high-pitched vocalisations when they are trapped by the sow. This gives the trapped piglet more chances of survival, since it will die by asphyxiation if its mother takes too long to realise what is occurring and stand up (Fig. 2).

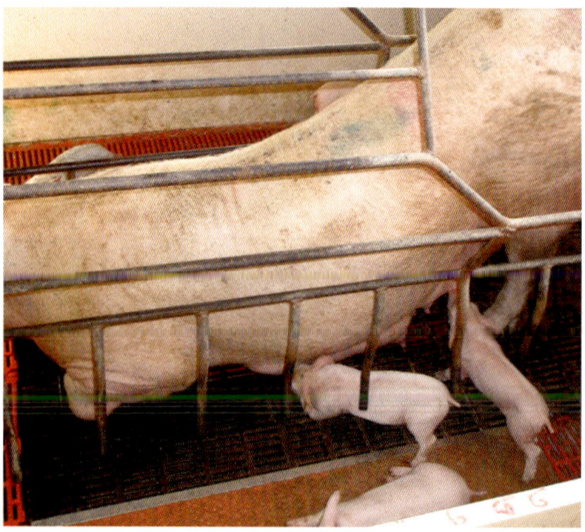

Figure 1 Sow lying down carefully in order not to crush her piglets.

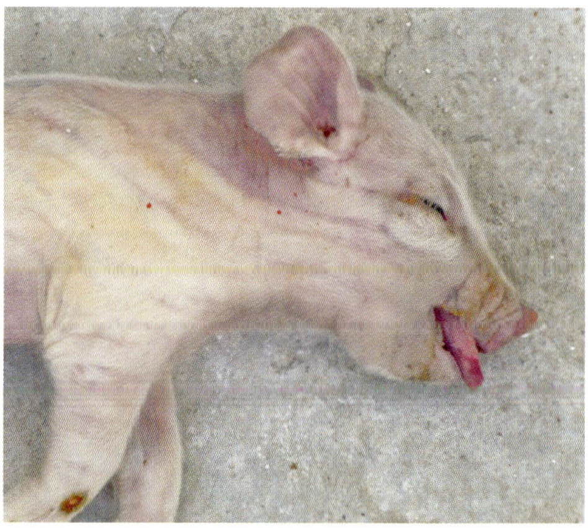

Figure 2 Piglet crushed by its mother. Skin lesions and cyanosis of the mucosae may be observed.

Sows need a very quiet environment to nurse their piglets properly and display appropriate maternal behaviour; any cause of stress (noises, unknown personnel, etc.) will make them fearful and anxious and may result in difficulties to nurse their litter and a reduction in their milk production.

The sows that display inappropriate behaviour should be identified so as to control them and euthanise them if necessary, especially on selection farms. The selection of sows for numerical productivity should be accompanied by new studies on behaviour to characterise mothering abilities and select females with good behaviour.

Weaning

Under natural conditions, weaning is a gradual process in all mammal species. As the offspring grow, their nutritional needs change and increase. Their mother's milk production is therefore insufficient to satisfy them. The offspring progressively get used to the solid foods their species requires.

In the case of sows, gradually and as lactation progresses, these may even reject nursing attempts by their piglets. In wild pigs, piglets make a slow transition from a diet exclusively based on milk to a diet with no milk until they become nutritionally independent from the sow at about 8 to 12 weeks of age. Other authors mention a longer process of up to 17 weeks.

The gradual process through which piglets change from one diet to another includes four phases.

1. **Hiding:** first week of lactation. The piglets remain isolated in the nest built by their mother and sporadically make excursions around it.
2. **Familiarising:** second and third week of lactation. The piglets leave the nest and follow the sow. They remain with the rest of the litter, but do not interact with the other piglets, or only very little. They start rooting in this phase.
3. **Integration and learning:** until the seventh week of lactation. The piglets increase their foraging behaviour and interact with other piglets from their social group. The sow leaves them alone for increasingly longer periods of time, the time interval between two nursing sessions increases and these are increasingly shorter.
4. **Independence:** until the seventeenth week of lactation, maximum. Nursing becomes increasingly less frequent until it ceases at some point. The piglets "function" independently as part of the extended social group. They feed on their own although they still sleep with the social group and their mother.

The interval between nursing cycles varies greatly. It lasts 40-60 minutes during the first week of lactation and then increases to 90 minutes between the second and fourth week. From the tenth week of lactation, the interval between two nursing sessions lasts 300 minutes.

Physiology of lactation

Mammary gland formation

The formation of the mammary glands from skin cells starts very early during foetal development. Before one month of gestation, it is already possible to observe the differentiation of the mammary lines, with thickenings that will eventually form the future teats; there will be as many as the number of mammary glands in the adult pig. On about day 70 of foetal life, each future mammary gland can be observed as a bud with an outer part that will form the teat, and an inner part that will give rise to the mammary ducts. These buds both develop into the lactiferous ducts and grow in a conical shape, so that they are raised from the skin surface, thereby forming the teat.

A rudimentary duct system with no gland tissue is already present when the piglets are born. Mammary glands remain inactive until puberty. At that moment and at the start of sexual maturity, they develop under the effect of ovarian hormones, and the non-glandular tissue starts to develop rapidly. The ducts form a very dense network, mainly of stroma.

Most of this development takes place from the second half of gestation (70-90 days), when the fat and connective tissue (stroma) is replaced by parenchyma (lobular-alveolar tissue). From day 90, the number of epithelial cells is highest and the mammary gland's secretory activity starts.

After farrowing, the increase in prolactin levels and decrease in oestrogen and progesterone levels lead to an increase in milk secretion. Nursing by the piglets and the action of oxytocin lead to the ejection of colostrum and milk.

Anatomical review of the mammary gland

The sow's mammary glands extend from the sternum to the inguinal region. They appear as raised areas with the shape of half spheres across the ventral region, each with its respective teat.

As shown in Figure 3, each gland has two totally independent duct systems; each system has a small cistern and a duct. The cistern or lactiferous sinus is an elliptical dilatation of the duct; its walls form numerous longitudinal folds, which close the passage to the lactiferous ducts hermetically. The cistern is communicated with the gland's internal wall through the ducts. The function of the ducts is to drain the milk located in the alveoli. Each mammary gland functions independently.

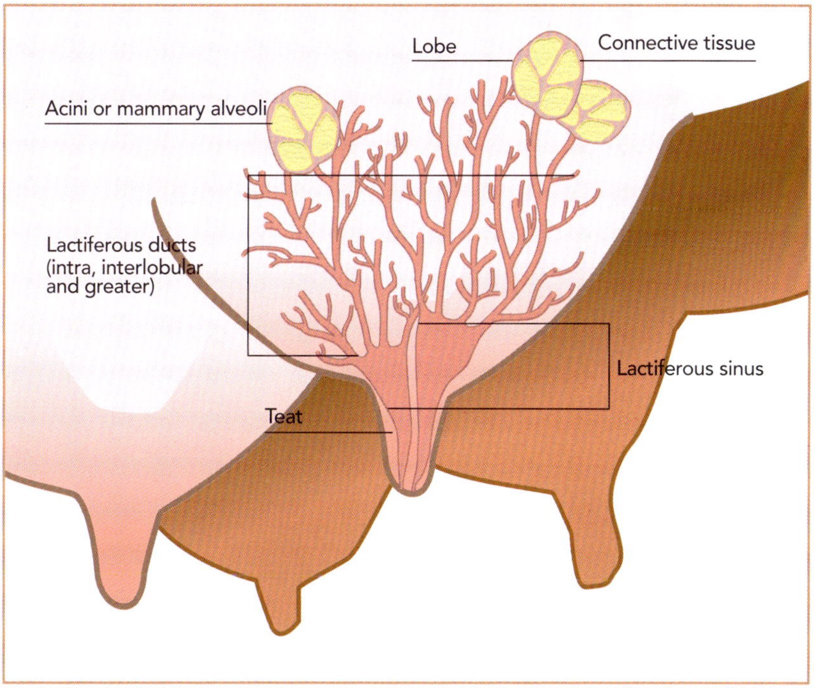

Figure 3 Structure of the mammary gland.

Number and type of teats

The sow's number of mammary glands varies depending on the breed; the average value is 10 teats for Iberian pig breeds, 10-12 for Duroc-Jersey breeds, 14-16 for Large White and Landrace breeds and 18 or more for Chinese breeds.

Genetic improvement has led to genetic lines of Large White and Landrace sows with 18 or more teats. The most advanced genetic selection programmes are currently working on selecting replacement gilts with a minimum of 14-16 functional teats.

Regarding the anatomical location of the mammary glands in sows, the first two pairs are usually thoracic, the last pair is inguinal and the other intermediate pairs are abdominal (Fig. 4). Mammary glands are located along the ventral median line (on the mammary ridges) and have some degree of bilateralism, although it is common to find a percentage of animals with an odd number of mammary glands.

Anatomical and physiological differences are responsible for variations in milk production. The anterior or thoracic mammary glands have a greater blood supply than the posterior ones (abdominal or inguinal) and therefore produce more milk. Not all the mammary glands are functional; it is common to find inverted or invaginated teats, which characteristically lack a glandular body and are shorter (17-30 % of sows have one or more inverted teats). These abnormal teats do not produce milk and their incidence varies according to authors.

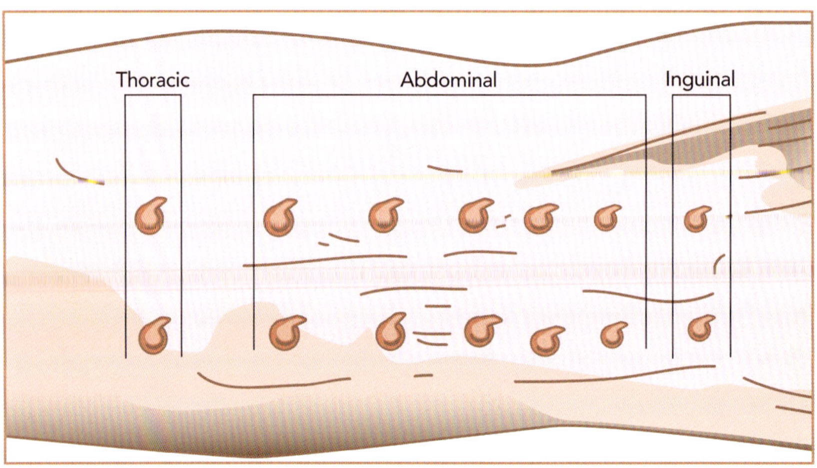

Figure 4 Number of mammary glands and anatomical distribution. Adapted from *Fallo lactacional de la cerda* (Barceló, J. and De Paz, X. , 2005).

Teats and mammary glands according to the sow's number of gestations or time of lactation

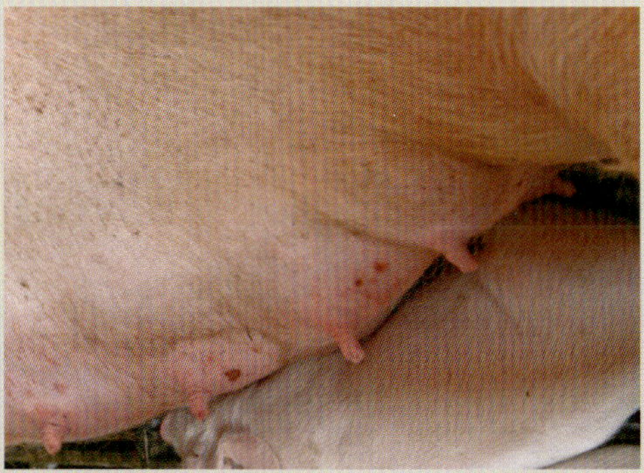

Figure 5 First-parity gilt.

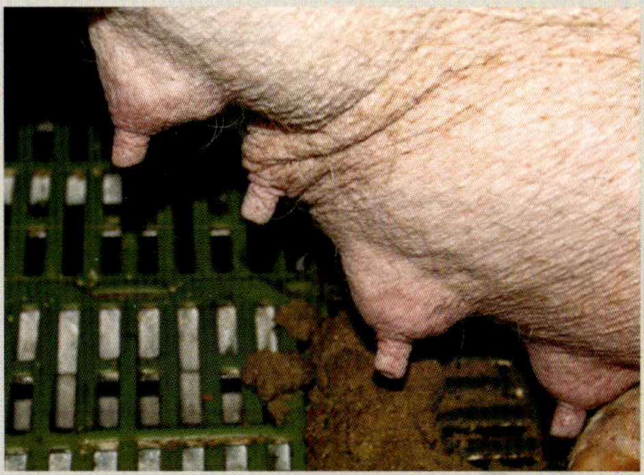

Figure 6 Multiparous sow.

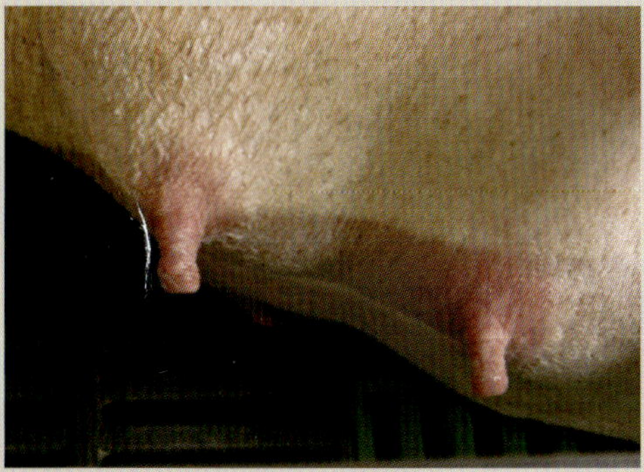

Figure 7 Ideal teats for nurse sows (long and thin).

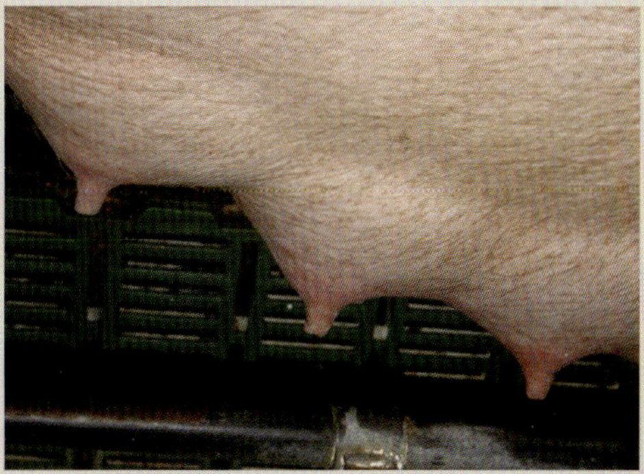

Figure 8 Before starting lactation.

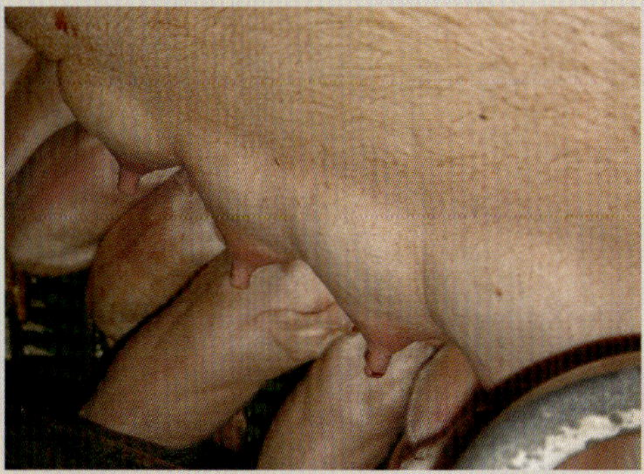

Figure 9 First week of lactation.

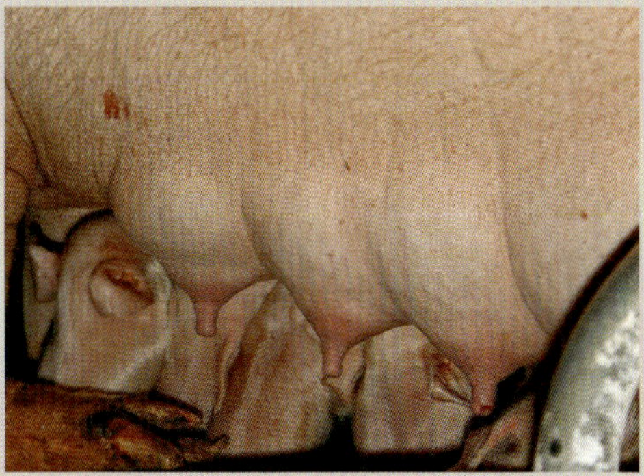

Figure 10 Late lactation.

Milk production depends on udder massaging and teat sucking by the corresponding piglet. If no piglet suckles from a teat, after three days without any stimulus, the mammary gland will undergo involution, which may become irreversible.

Endocrinology of lactation

The mammary glands experience continuous structural and functional changes related to the sow's age (mainly puberty), the cycle phase (follicular or luteal) and her physiological stage: gestation, lactation or weaning.

Every year, the sow's mammary glands undergo 2.3-2.5 cycles of development, lactation and mammary involution. Mammary gland development in each lactation has an influence on the glands' production and functionality in the next lactation.

The lactation period has two independent phases: lactogenesis or milk formation, mainly regulated by prolactin; and milk ejection or let-down, regulated essentially by oxytocin.

Lactogenesis

In the gestating sow, progesterone levels start to decrease from the second or third week before farrowing, although the reduction is more marked in the last two days. This decrease in progesterone levels induces a rise in prolactin levels and therefore, an increase in the size of the mammary glands, which grow mainly in the last three weeks of gestation and reach their maximum development in the three or four days previous to farrowing. A discharge of serous fluid through the teats is observed 48 hours before farrowing and the sow starts to secrete colostrum 24 hours before giving birth to her piglets.

Lactogenesis is divided into a secretory phase, during which colostrum and milk secretion starts, and a second phase of galactopoiesis, during which milk production is maintained throughout the whole lactation period until weaning. A good start to milk production is essential for a good lactation.

Mammary stimulation by a vigorous litter leads to an increase in prolactin levels and enhances milk production.

Maintenance of lactation (galactopoiesis)

The activity of the pituitary gland is essential for the maintenance of lactation and for milk secretion to begin. The continued production of prolactin is essential during the whole lactation period. The suckling stimulus of the piglets keeps prolactin levels high, which prolongs lactation and anoestrus in the sow.

If, for any reason, the suckling stimulus becomes weaker (partial weaning or nurse sows with very small piglets or piglets that do not nurse enough), the sow may come in heat even during lactation.

Milk ejection

The oxytocin released through the hypothalamic-pituitary axis causes milk ejection, or let-down, while the piglet is nursing. The production of this hormone is conditioned by a neurohormonal reflex caused by udder massaging and teat sucking by the piglets. The peripheral tactile information at the level of the mammary glands is transmitted through the nerves to the hypothalamic-pituitary axis, which induces the release of oxytocin to the bloodstream. The hormone reaches the mammary glands, where it causes the contraction of the myoepithelial cells and the emptying of the alveoli. The milk produced passes to the lactiferous ducts and comes out from the teat when the piglets are nursing.

Lactation curve and milk production

A sow's milk production mainly depends on her piglets' vigour when sucking the milk from the mammary glands, and varies in function of the litter size, number of lactations, genetic line and feeding during the gestation phase and above all during lactation.

The best way to calculate a sow's milk production is to monitor the weight of her piglets, although the data obtained this way may be partly erroneous. Some studies have established that every kg of weight gained by a piglet is equivalent to four litres of milk. Therefore, a sow that weans 11 piglets with an average weight of 6.4 kg after 22 days and with a birth weight of 1.4 kg produces 220 litres of milk during her lactation; that is to say, an average of ten litres a day. In another study (2009), Collell mentions maximum productions of up to 12 litres a day (Fig. 11). Nowadays, these figures are even exceeded in some sows with productive peaks of 14 or more litres a day.

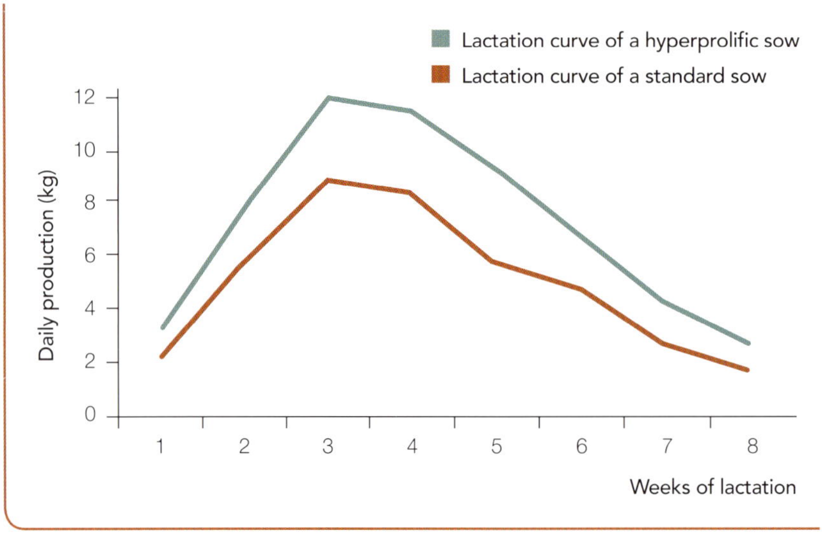

Figure 11 Lactation curves of a standard sow and a hyperprolific sow.

Phases of nursing

Based on piglet behaviour, there are three phases during a nursing bout (Fig. 12).

- **First phase:** very vigorous previous mammary massage that stimulates oxytocin production. The piglets compete with each other and squeal. The sow grunts and calls her piglets, which coincides with the elimination of oxytocin. This phase lasts between 1 and 3 minutes.
- **Second phase:** known as the milk ingestion or nutritive phase. When they hear the sow's signal, the piglets remain quiet and suckle at the teat waiting for the milk to let down. As soon as it comes out, the piglets drink it very quickly (Fig. 12). This phase only lasts between 10 and 20 seconds. In this phase, oxytocin causes the contraction of the myoepithelial cells of the mammary alveoli and milk let-down occurs.
- **Third phase:** it includes the massage of the mammary glands after milk ejection. After ingesting the milk, the piglets massage the mammary glands, albeit in a less vigorous manner, and the sow becomes quiet and grunts softly.

Three stages may also be distinguished depending on whether the initiator of the nursing bout is the sow or the piglets:

- During the first ten days of life of the piglets, in 60-80 % of cases, the sow is responsible for the stimulation of nursing, as she produces more milk than the amount her piglets are able to ingest.

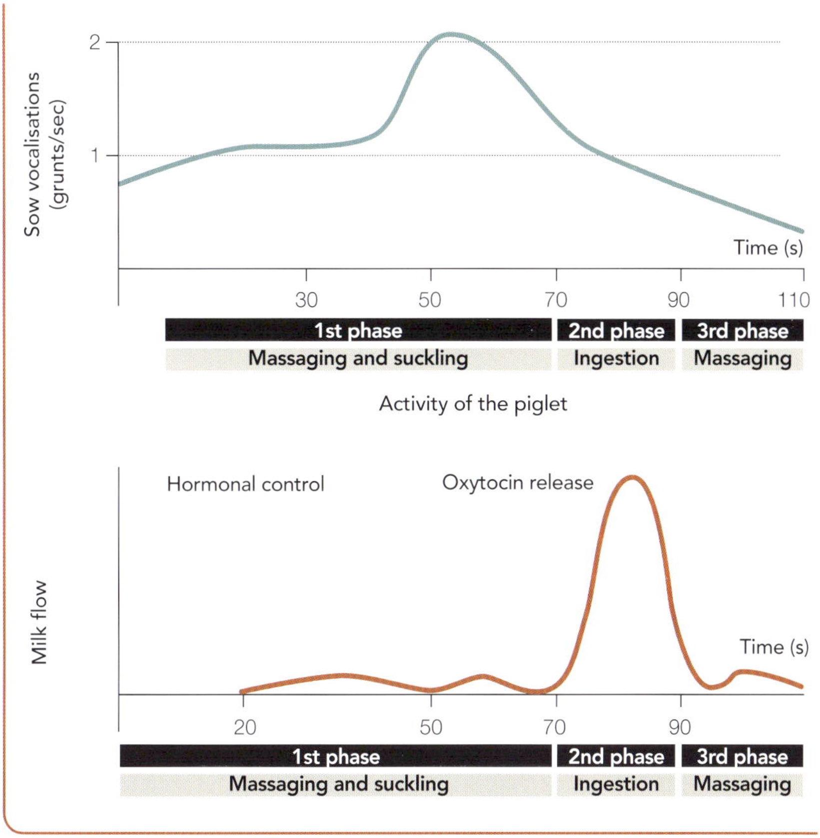

Figure 12 Lactation curves. Adapted from Whittemore, C. T. *The science and practice of pig production*. Harlow Scientific and Technical Editions, Arlington, 1993.

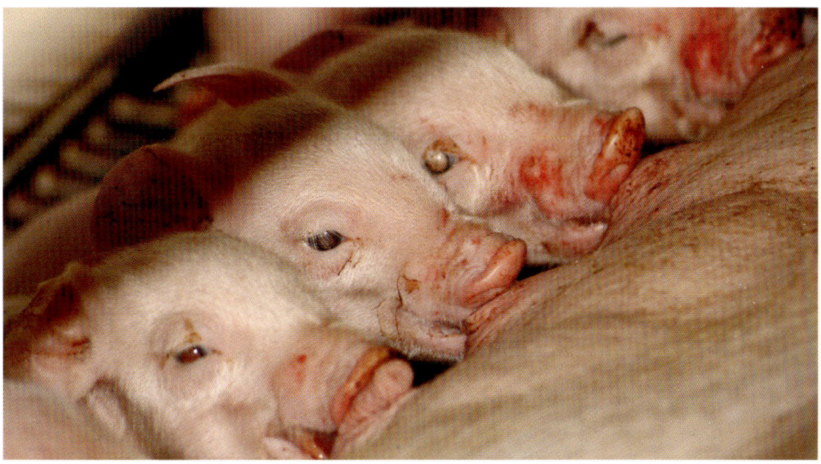

Figure 13 Piglets in the second phase of nursing: milk ingestion or nutritive phase.

- From day 30 of lactation, piglets require more milk and therefore stimulate nursing, as the sow is not able to produce enough milk for the whole litter.
- During the litter's first 10-30 days of life, it is unclear whether nursing is sitmulated by the sow or by her piglets.

Composition of colostrum

Colostrum is the sow's first mammary secretion after farrowing. It has two essential characteristics: it is very rich in maternal antibodies (immunoglobulins) and has a high nutritional value, which is indispensable to make up for the low energy reserves with which piglets are born, so they do not lose their body temperature during their first hours of life. In comparison with milk, colostrum is poorer in fat and lactose, but richer in proteins (immunoglobulins) (Table 1).

Composition differences (g/kg)	Colostrum	Milk
Water	700	800
Fat	70	90
Lactose	25	50
Proteins	200	55
Ashes	5	5

Table 1 Composition differences between colostrum and milk (g/kg). From Whittemore, C. T. *The science and practice of pig production*. Harlow Scientific and Technical Editions, Arlington, 1993.

Piglets are very vulnerable at birth and have no humoral immunity or acquired antibodies, as there is no mother-foetus placental transfer of antibodies. Antibodies are molecules incapable of passing through the placental barrier; piglets are therefore born without any antibodies and need them to be transmitted by their mother through colostrum after birth (indispensable for their survival). It is very important for piglets to receive antibodies during their first hours of life, as their intestinal mucosa is still permeable to these molecules immediately after birth. However, after the first few hours of life, this permeability decreases, thereby preventing antibodies from passing through the intestinal wall. If a piglet does not receive maternal antibodies, it may become very susceptible to any kind of infections.

Colostrum stimulates the development of the piglet's digestive tract. Furthermore, it is highly digestible, but also slightly laxative, which allows the fast elimination of excrement from the digestive tract. The total colostrum production is highly variable (from 2 to 6 litres) and lasts from farrowing to approximately 18-24 hours after the start of lactation (Fig. 14). At each ejection, 30-100 ml are produced. Piglets obtain colostrum easily every 10-20 seconds without barely massaging the mammary glands.

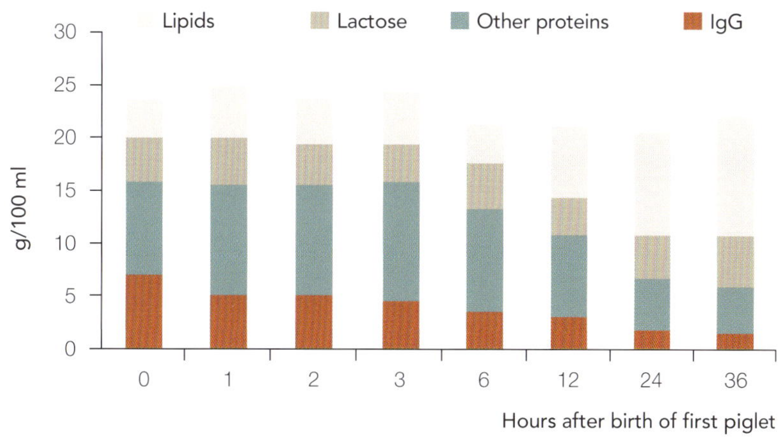

Figure 14 Composition of colostrum and evolution after birth. Adapted from Le Dividich, INRA, March 2006.

Composition of milk

The function of the sow's milk is to feed her litter; it is vital for the survival of the piglets in their first weeks of life.

The main characteristics of milk are:

- High palatability: increases intake and favours the development of the digestive tract.
- High digestibility of its nutrients (mainly fat and casein): adapted to early ages. Casein provides the calcium necessary for bone growth.
- High lactose content: favours the proliferation of saprophytic bacteria such as *Lactobacillus*, in addition to contributing to a reduction of the stomach pH as lactose is transformed into lactic acid.
- High growth factor, vitamin and mineral content.

A sow secretes milk at frequent intervals and milk secretion is therefore adapted to the digestive capacity of piglets in the first few days. The composition of milk and colostrum is very different with regard to proteins, lactose and antibodies, as can be seen in Table 1.

Physiology of the suckling piglet

Birth-to-weaning mortality

The porcine species is characterised by a high mortality rate, due to the physiology of piglets, as they are born with very marked physiological deficiencies. This hinders their adaptation to their new environment during their first 24-72 hours of life.

The low birth weight of piglets in comparison with their adult weight (a little more than 1 %), the fact that they are born without a protective layer of hair and with a very thin layer of subcutaneous fat, as well as the fact that they barely have energy reserves to draw on at birth are some of their main physiological deficiencies. In addition, piglets have a greater relative body surface than adult pigs. All these circumstances lead to a low body thermal insulation, which is exacerbated by the fact that they do not have a mature thermoregulation system at the time of birth. All this contributes to a considerable number of deaths due to hypothermia.

According to reference data from the data bank on Spanish pig production (BDporc, 2013), the average mortality rate from birth to weaning in 2013 was 12.14 % for a sample of more than 600,000 sows. On farms with excellent management practices, this figure may be reduced to 4-5 %.

The different mortality rates from birth to weaning depend on:

- Factors associated with the piglet such as birth weight, immunity level, breed and genetics.
- Factors associated with the sow such as number of farrowings, weight, maternal behaviour, milk production and litter size.
- Factors associated with the environment and production systems such as facilities, workforce, husbandry practices, feeding and ambient temperature.

Between 70 % and 80 % of deaths in piglets in the farrowing room occur during their first three days of life.

Hierarchy

Dominant-subordinate relationships are described in almost all groups of animals. The concept of dominance involves an asymmetric relationship between two individuals, which is mainly manifested in two ways: the subordinate receives most aggressions, and when competing for the same resource (for example, the best thoracic teats), it is the dominant individual that obtains access to it in most cases.

During the first days postpartum, piglets compete with each other to have access to a specific teat.

During their first three days of life, piglets already compete for the best teats and establish a hierarchical order that will determine their access to these teats (Figs. 15 and 16). In a simplified manner, this competition process takes place in four phases:

1. **Teat seeking** starts immediately after birth, when the newborn piglet walks around the sow and ends when the first teat is located.
2. **Teat sampling** then takes places; the piglet moves from teat to teat and starts trying to move other littermates from their positions.
3. The next phase is **teat defence**. Once the piglet has chosen a teat, it does not leave it. It pulls and presses on it and defends it aggressively by biting and pushing with its body and nose those that try to get to the teat. This fighting behaviour decreases as hours pass by and disappears once a hierarchy has been established, according to which a piglet will always suckle at the same teat or at the most at the same pair of teats. Of course, the strongest piglets choose the teats that produce more milk.
4. When a piglet has chosen a teat, it will suckle at it throughout the whole lactation period. This is called the **maintenance phase**. When using cross-fostering techniques or nurse sows, it is very important to take each position into account, in order to avoid new fights to establish a new hierarchical order.

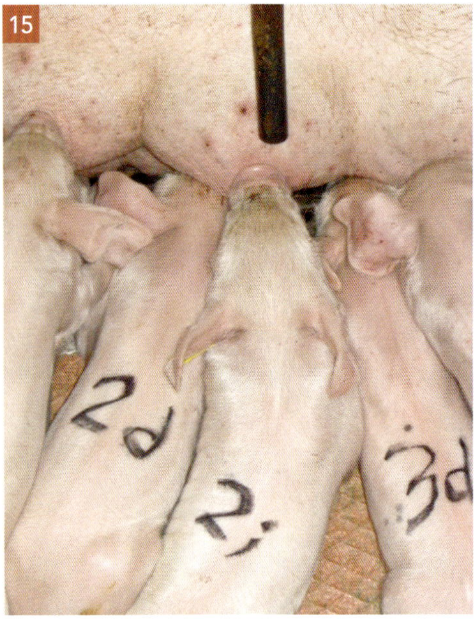

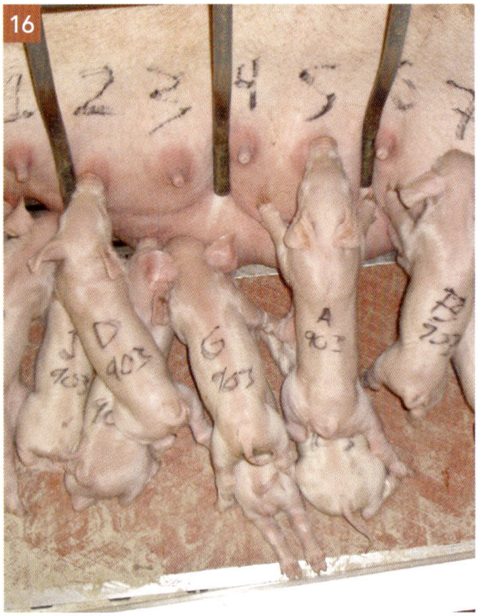

Figures 15 and 16 Images of an experiment carried out by the authors in which the teats and piglets were numbered to check whether these always suckled at the same teat.

Pigs are very hierarchical animals. A very strict hierarchy is established almost from birth and conditions behaviour patterns and management practices during lactation and subsequently throughout their whole adult life.

Play

Piglets often play, although they dedicate most of their daily activity to sleeping and resting (about 80 % of their time) and the rest to eating, by nursing approximately every hour.

Although some authors do not agree with this idea, play does not seem to have a specific function, but this does not mean that it does not have a positive influence on the individual's development. It seems that play is a learning or training method for adult life, although there is not enough experimental data available to confirm this fact. On the other hand, some hypotheses claim that play at a young age has long-term effects on the response to stress in adult life, so that the piglets that play a lot may suffer from less stress in the future. Play is an indicator of welfare and health; sick piglets do not play.

Physiology of weaning

Hormonal changes in the sow

The high progesterone levels maintained during the whole gestation period stimulate mammary gland development, especially from days 70-90 since fertilisation (this is when the udders develop most) while inhibiting lactogenesis at the same time.

After farrowing, progesterone levels decrease and prolactin is released by the pituitary gland. The pituitary gland is essential for the maintenance of lactation and for milk secretion to begin. The continuous suckling stimulus by the piglets ensures prolactin levels remain high, as well as galactopoietic hormones (also secreted by the pituitary gland), which are responsible for the maintenance of lactation.

Age at weaning

In the main pig-producing countries, the age at weaning has progressively been reduced for the last 30 years, due to the continuous pressure of the pig industry to improve its efficiency. In a majority of the most efficient countries in pig production, the average age at weaning is between 21 and 24 days.

With the emergence of PRRS (porcine reproductive and respiratory syndrome) and pig production by phases, the average age at weaning was considerably reduced, to 18-20 days, as sows were not weaned at more than 21 days of lactation for sanitary reasons. However, nowadays, tendencies have changed with the appearance of hyperprolific lines and the introduction of fostering techniques for large numbers of piglets. The tendency is therefore to increase the age at weaning to 28 days, so piglets can be weaned with an appropriate weight and uterine involution is optimal.

Weight at weaning and growth curve

Weight at weaning depends essentially on the age of the piglet at that time and on the sow's milk production capacity. It also depends on the piglet's birth weight and on whether it has suffered from any health problems (*E.coli* diarrhoea, essentially) or environmental problems (low temperature, draughts, etc.), especially in its first days of life.

The authors' recommendation is to not wean piglets under 7 kg of live weight or less than 24-25 days of life, to ensure their future development and perfect uterine involution.

Piglets grow very fast when they are in the farrowing unit. In four weeks, they almost multiply their initial weight by five; as a result, piglets with birth weights of 1.450 kg can reach average weights of more than 8 kg in 28 days (Fig. 17).

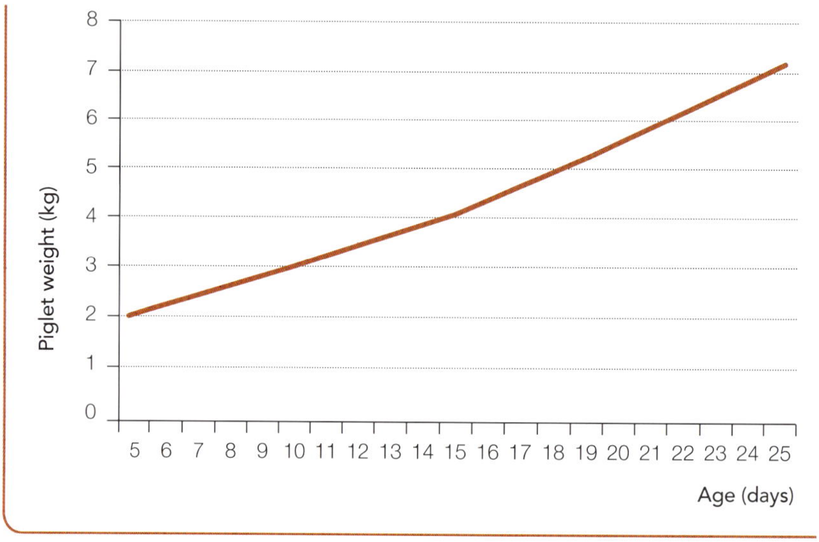

Figure 17 Growth curve of a piglet between 5 and 25 days of age. The average weight varies between 5-6 kg with piglets weaned at 21 days; and 7-9 kg with piglets weaned at 28 days.

Newly weaned piglets lose more than 10 % of their total weight during the first two days post-weaning.

Weaning and stress in the piglet

At weaning, piglets face three great challenges:

1. The first challenge corresponds to the significant **changes in the composition of their food and how it is supplied**, as they change from a liquid diet provided in cycles and based on milk (20 % dry matter), with dry matter rich in proteins (30 %), fat (40 %) and lactose (25 %), but no starch; to a new more abundant diet fed ad libitum and composed of ingredients they have not tasted yet and in dry form (88 % of dry matter). As a result, their digestive tract undergoes an important transition from the digestion of fat to that of complex carbohydrates.
2. The second challenge that piglets must face are the **changes in the physical and environmental conditions**. They are used to living in farrowing pens with their mother and littermates and have to learn to live without their mother and usually to share their space with more piglets.
3. The third challenge is the **psychological stress** of being transferred to a different location and mixed with other animals (which often includes transport to other farms), which gives rise to numerous fights in order to reestablish the strong social hierarchy of piglets.

The result of all these changes is usually that newly weaned piglets lose a considerable amount of weight –more than 10 % their total weight– on the first two days after weaning. They do not recover their usual intake (similar to their intake of milk plus the starter feed they were fed during the lactation period) until day 7 post-weaning.

The separation of a piglet from its mother is accompanied by characteristic, loud grunts or calls by the sow immediately after weaning. The frequency of these calls is higher at the beginning and in litters weaned of three or fewer weeks of age.

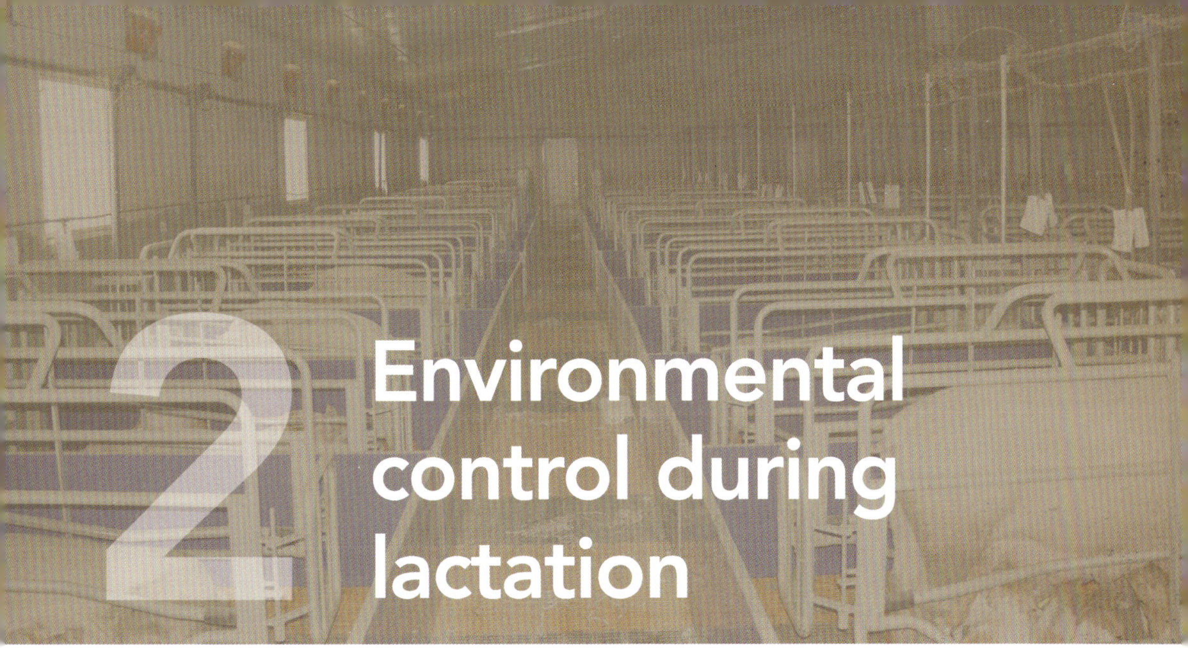

2 Environmental control during lactation

Introduction

The energy costs of farms are very likely to keep increasing in the future, despite the use of renewable energies and the application of the new technologies currently being developed. This factor may affect competitiveness among operations in the same country and among the different pork-producing countries. The use of automated environmental control systems in farrowing units is therefore essential to ensure the animals on the farm express their maximum productive potential effectively and energy costs are reduced to a minimum.

Moreover, it should be remembered that the insulation capacity of the roof and exterior walls of farrowing units is a key factor to avoid heat losses in winter, and excess heat in summer.

Keys to a good environmental control

The objective is to provide excellent environmental comfort to both the sows and their piglets. First of all, the animals' thermal comfort requirements should be met with the help of heating and cooling systems when necessary, without neglecting air renewal in the rooms in order to provide, by means of ventilation systems, the oxygen required and eliminate toxic and harmful gases as well as any excess humidity. This may seem simple at first but it is a very complex task in practice, since the thermal comfort requirements of sows are very different from those of piglets, especially newborn piglets.

Moreover, measuring devices can provide us with data about the temperature in the room and creep areas, the air intake velocity in the room, the relative humidity levels..., but they do not offer information about the thermal comfort felt by the animals. In piglets, this sensation significantly varies depending on the type of flooring (fully slatted floors or solid floors in creep areas), the heating system used (underfloor heating or heat lamps), the air velocity at their height, etc. These factors are similar for sows (type of flooring, proximity of the heat source to their head, etc.).

It is thus crucial to calculate their environmental requirements accurately and ensure the heating, cooling and ventilation systems necessary are well-designed based on the type of farrowing room and its dimensions, as well as on the weather conditions of the geographical area where the farm is located. In addition, some routine control systems should also be established to guarantee the environmental comfort of the animals over time.

Figure 1 Comfort, the number 1 objective. Adapted from Escobet, J. *Climatización de la transición*, 2013.

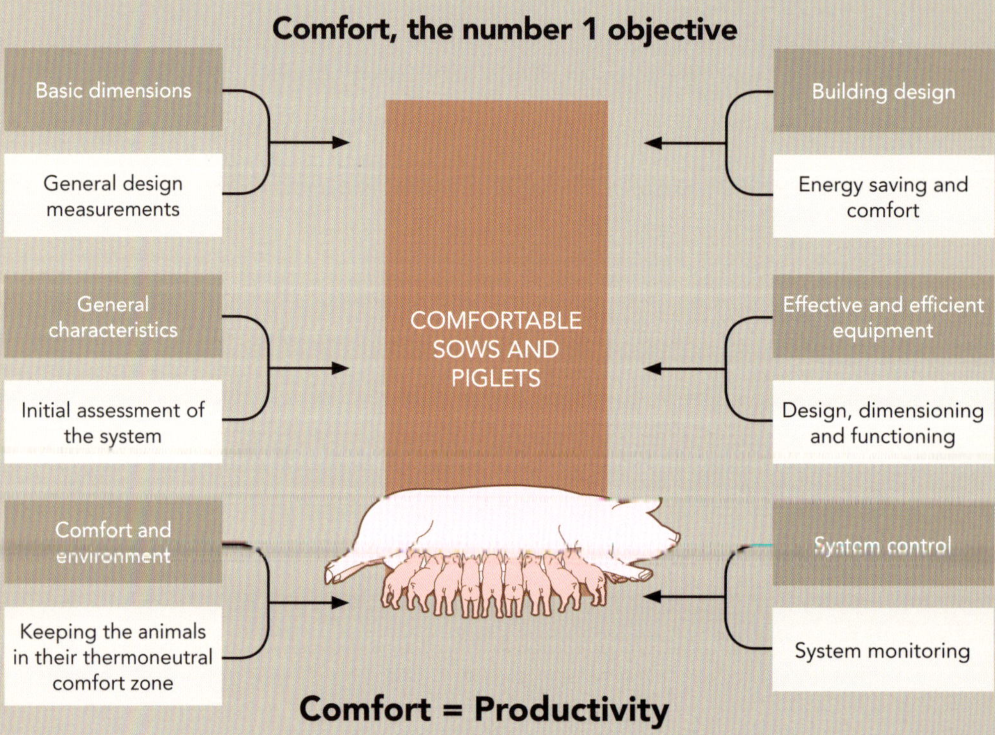

Thermal comfort in the farrowing unit

Pigs are homeothermic animals; however, unlike human beings and other animals, they barely sweat. They regulate their temperature by increasing their respiratory rate (what is known as panting) in order to lose heat, or by increasing their feed intake and metabolism when they are cold to maintain their body temperature. By increasing their activity (moving, shivering...), they can enhance their production of heat. All these systems consume a lot of energy, and this factor is negatively correlated with performance parameters.

Homeothermic animals exchange heat with the environment through several mechanisms:

- **Conduction:** this occurs when there is an energy exchange between the animal and the surfaces with which it is in contact. An example of this is when a sow is hot and lies down on her side on the farrowing room floor, thereby increasing her contact surface and losing this excess heat. Conversely, if she is cold, she will lie down on her abdomen or sit down on her legs to reduce the contact surface. The heat transfer characteristics of materials are very important to help sows thermoregulate themselves. Placing cast iron under the sows in the farrowing rooms is therefore recommended.
- **Convection:** this term refers to the heat exchange that takes place between an animal's surface and the air that surrounds it. This explains why it is essential to ensure the ambient temperature is in accordance with the animals' comfort temperature. Ventilation systems to control air flows are the key to this mechanism. Ventilation tends to be increased in summer, so that there is a good air flow at the height of the sows in order for them to exchange more heat with the environment; while in winter, when temperatures are very low, ventilation is reduced to avoid strong air draughts above the animals.
- **Radiation:** animals emit electromagnetic waves that result from heat production by their organism. These waves travel to the materials that surround the sows. These absorb part of the waves and transform them again into heat. When it is cold and ventilation rates are low, this type of exchange is almost as significant as that resulting from convection.
- **Evaporation:** it is the mechanism used by sows when the ambient temperature is high and there is little difference between the temperature of their body surface and that of the environment. Sows increase their respiratory rate and, as a result, the diffusion of water vapour through panting. This system is more efficient when the relative humidity levels in the environment are low.

Thermal comfort of the sow

All the mechanisms previously described require energy expenditure for the production or reduction of body heat. The objective is an environmental temperature in the rooms that can, to the extent possible, maintain the sows within their **thermal comfort zone (TCZ)**, with a minimum energy consumption for thermoregulation and thus a better productive efficiency (Fig. 2).

> When sows do not use up their energy to produce heat or lower their body temperature, they are in their **thermoneutral zone (TNZ).**

In winter (cold season)

When the ambient temperature in the farrowing rooms falls below a certain level, the sows increase their feed intake and their basal metabolic rate to produce heat and maintain their body temperature. When this mechanism is activated, it is said that their **lower critical temperature (LCT)** has been reached.

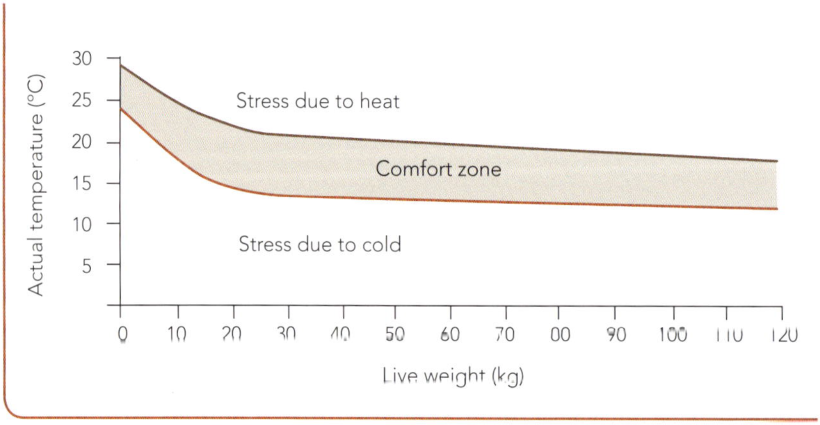

Figure 2 Evolution of comfort temperatures in pigs according to their live weight. Adapted from McFarlane, J. Temperatura efectiva del entorno y confort. *Suis*, 2004.

If this only occurs sporadically on very cold winter days, the installation of an extra heating system in the farrowing unit is not profitable. Nevertheless, in geographical areas where extremely low temperatures can be reached, the installation of systems to provide extra heat to the rooms is necessary. The systems usually used include unit heaters, hot-water radiators in the unit's main corridor or delta pipes next to the entrance to the rooms.

Energy expenses will always be lower than the costs resulting from the extra intake of feed. The most dangerous situation occurs when a sow draws on her fat reserves during lactation to produce heat, thereby reducing her litter's development and her future performance levels.

In summer (warm season)

When the ambient temperature in the rooms exceeds a certain level, the sows start to activate their mechanisms of defence. They basically increase their respiratory rate and sweat in order to lose heat through evaporation, in an attempt to maintain their body temperature. At that moment, it is said that they have reached their **evaporative critical temperature (ECT)**.

If the ambient temperature continues to increase, there is a point when the sows are no longer able to prevent their body temperature from increasing. This point is called the **upper critical temperature (UCT)**. From this point, body temperature rises rapidly, which may cause death of the animals (Fig. 3).

Aspects to be considered to improve thermal comfort

- **Insulation of the roof and exterior walls.** The greater the variation range between the minimum and maximum outside temperature, the more important the level of insulation of the farrowing unit enclosures. A good calculation and choice of materials to be installed when designing the unit will lead to considerable savings in the future energy consumption to maintain a comfortable temperature in the rooms.
- **Regulation of the ventilation systems.** Excess ventilation on days of extreme cold should be avoided. Measuring equipments should be regularly inspected (cleanliness of the sensors, of the air inlets...).
- **Doors, windows, chimneys, etc. should seal tightly.** This is essential to avoid cold air coming from outside.

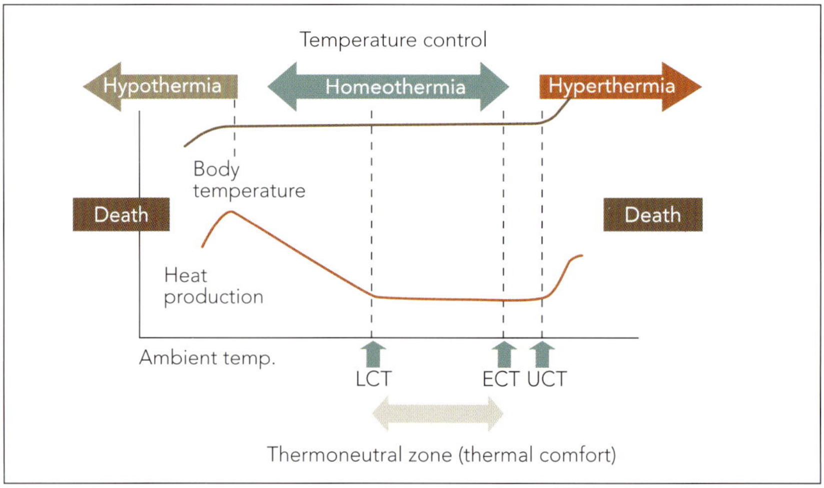

Figure 3 Regulation of body temperature. Adapted from Collell, M. *Manejo del calor*, 2009.

Systems used to guarantee the thermal comfort of sows

When sows are hot, they become stressed, reduce their feed intake and draw on their body reserves to maintain milk production. Paradoxically, their milk production drops dramatically and the viability and weight at weaning of their litters are significantly reduced. Moreover, the body condition of the piglets at weaning worsens and the sows' performance in their next reproductive cycle is compromised (poor heat signs, lower ovulation rate, higher repeat rates, embryonic deaths...).

For each degree above 23 °C (ECT), sows reduce their feed intake by 170 g (between 100 and 300 g). Their milk production and the weaning weight of their litter also go down and their body condition worsens.

As a result, it is indispensable to install and use cooling systems in farrowing units to reduce the ambient temperature in the rooms in the hot season. These cooling systems work by mixing outside air, which is not saturated with water vapour, with liquid water or water mist. The partial pressure difference between the air and the water causes a transfer of water to the air in the form of vapour, thereby reducing the temperature of the air drawn in the room. This technique is called "evaporative cooling" and works better when the ambient relative humidity levels are low. The most commonly used cooling systems on swine operations are high-pressure fogging systems and cooling pads.

High-pressure fogging systems

The system consists of a high-pressure pump and pipes (preferably made of stainless steel) which are fitted with special nozzles, also made of stainless steel, which spray water in the form of very fine droplets. These remain suspended in the air so that the outside air entering the room evaporates them when it comes in contact with the "cloud" formed, thereby increasing the relative humidity and reducing the temperature (Fig. 4).

It is important to precisely calculate the pressure, water flow, number of nozzles required and the distance between them in order to ensure that all the water evaporates before reaching the floor. In large farrowing rooms, two parallel rows may be installed, but these have to be at a sufficient distance from one another to prevent the droplets sprayed from a line to reach those sprayed from the other, as they would otherwise fuse and become larger, which would make them fall to the ground. The same occurs with the distance between the nozzles of a same row.

Efficacy depends on the size of the droplets, which is determined by the pressure of the water and the diameter of the nozzle. Droplets with a diameter of 40 to 100 µm at a pressure of 300 to 600 kPa are usually used in farrowing facilities, with a water flow of 4-8 litres per hour.

The pipes are installed close to the air inlets in the rooms and as high as possible. They are placed depending on the height at which these inlets are located (Fig. 5).

Figure 4 High-pressure fogging system. From Blanes-Vidal, V. and Torres, A. G. Diseño y evaluación de la calefacción y de la refrigeración. In: Forcada, F. et al. *Ganado porcino. Diseño de alojamientos e instalaciones.* Zaragoza: Servet, 2009.

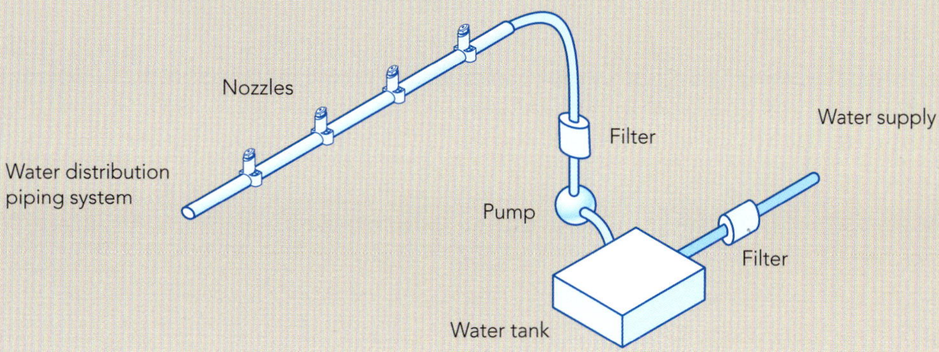

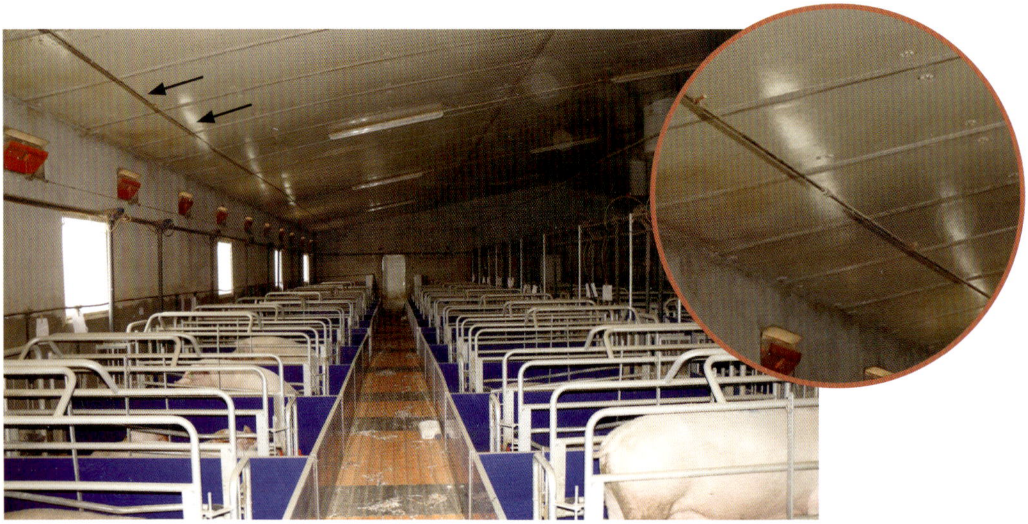

Figure 5 High-pressure fogging system above the windows.

The duration of use can be set based on the temperature in the rooms. As the temperature rises, the "on" periods become longer, and alternate with "off" periods which are automatically adjusted.

Regular inspection and proper maintenance of the system are essential (cleaning of nozzles, control of the pressure...) to avoid efficacy losses. Filters are necessary to eliminate impurities from the water as it enters the high-pressure pump to avoid dirt from accumulating in the nozzles. In places where water is very hard, a water softener should be installed (salt, acid injection or others). If this is not done, calcium rapidly clogs the openings of the nozzles.

Cooling pads

These pads are placed at the air inlets in the unit's corridor (exterior walls or in the roof) or directly at the air inlets in the rooms depending on how these and the ventilation systems are designed (Figs. 6 and 7). The piping system is usually made of stainless steel or PVC and forms a circuit which is connected to a tank. There may be one tank per pad or (usually) one single tank for all the pads. The pipes have holes placed above the pads so that a curtain of water flows through them. The water is collected at the bottom of the pads and pumped back to the tank.

As with the previous system, as the hot air comes in contact with the damp pad, it collects moisture and cools down through evaporative cooling.

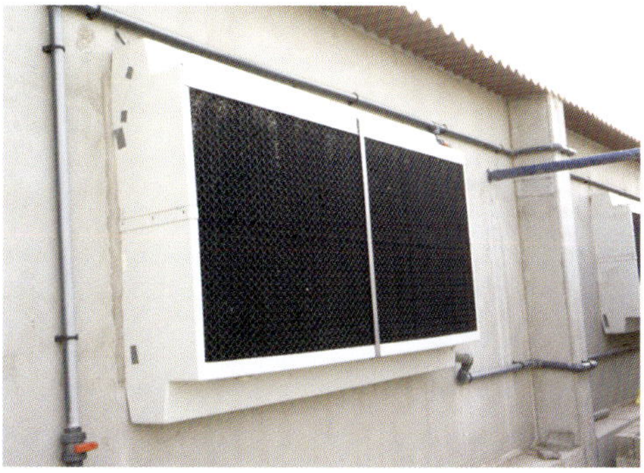

Figure 6 Evaporative cooling pads on an exterior wall.

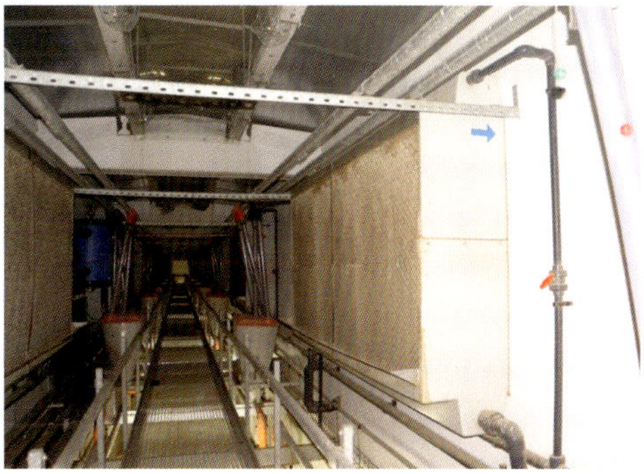

Figure 7 Evaporative cooling pads on the ceiling of the aisle.

The most commonly used pads are those made of chemically treated cellulose, but other materials are also available, such as fibreglass, PVC, wood shavings, aluminium, etc. The efficacy of a pad depends on its thickness and on the velocity of air as it passes through it. To achieve an optimal performance, the whole surface of the pad should be damp to increase the volume of cooled air that is drawn into the rooms through the suction effect from the exhaust fans. Depending on the thickness of the pads, the outside air takes a shorter or longer period of time to pass through them. This increases or reduces the contact time with water and therefore achieves higher or lower performance levels. Very thick pads may increase resistance to the passage of air and require the installation of more powerful fans in the rooms, thereby increasing acquisition costs as well as energy costs as a result of a higher consumption.

Air velocity should also be accurately calculated, since if the air goes through the pads very slowly, no turbulences are generated and little air comes in contact with the water and cools down. Conversely, if air velocity is too high, the air drawn in only comes in contact with the water for a short period of time and does not cool down sufficiently (Table 1).

In practice, the most commonly used pads are those made of chemically treated cellulose with a thickness of 10 to 15 cm and a maximum air velocity of 1.25 to 1.75 m/s (depending on their thickness). The width and height of the pads also vary greatly depending on the air conditioning system designs, but they should always guarantee a uniform air flow. When determining the dimension of the pads, all the variables already mentioned are calculated and, including under optimal conditions, the calculations should be carried out with an average performance of

Table 1 Average air velocity, minimum water flow and minimum capacity of the water tank recommended. From Blanes-Vidal, V. and y Torres, A. G. Diseño y evaluación de la calefacción y de la refrigeración. In: Forcada, F. et al. *Ganado porcino. Diseño de alojamientos e instalaciones.* Zaragoza: Servet, 2009.

Material and thickness of the pad	Average air velocity through the pad (m/s)	Minimum water flow per horizontal metre of pad (l/min and m)	Minimum capacity of the water tank per m^2 of pad (l/m^2)
Wood shavings (poplar) Pad thickness: from 5 to 10 cm	0.75	5	20
Chemically treated cellulose Pad thickness 10 cm	1.25	6	30
Chemically treated cellulose Pad thickness 15 cm	1.75	10	40

about 80 %. This will ensure the pads will still be mostly effective when weather conditions are adverse due to high heat or humidity levels, etc. (Table 2).

As with the previous system, proper maintenance of the pads, pumps and piping system is essential to ensure they keep functioning correctly and to avoid losses of efficacy throughout time. Filters and, where appropriate, a water softening system should be installed. The accumulation of impurities and calcium in the pads reduces their performance. In addition, for evaporative cooling systems to work properly, they should be perfectly synchronised with the other environmental control systems installed on the farm.

Table 2 Decrease in the temperature of the incoming air by means of evaporative cooling pads (80 % performance). From Blanes-Vidal, V. and Torres, A. G. Diseño y evaluación de la calefacción y de la refrigeración. In: Forcada, F. et al. *Ganado porcino. Diseño de alojamientos e instalaciones.* Zaragoza: Servet, 2009.

	OUTSIDE RELATIVE HUMIDITY (%)							
	35				50			
Outside temperature (°C)	25	30	35	40	25	30	35	40
Decrease in the temperature of the incoming air (°C)	-8.5	-10	-11.5	-12.5	-6	-7	-7.5	-8.5

The choice of one system or another depends on the geographical area (environmental humidity, temperature...) and design of the ventilation system, as well as on how it is controlled. On modern facilities, a sensor to measure the relative humidity of the rooms is even installed so that, when it reaches 75-80%, the cooling systems turn off until this value goes down. In the same way, environmental control devices automatically turn on the cooling systems when, through different measurements, they detect that the temperature in the rooms is above a set value. They are usually programmed to start functioning when the ambient temperature in the room exceeds 25-26 °C or when the outside temperature is above 28-30 °C.

Moreover, the control systems have an acceleration curve that gradually increases the volume of air in contact with the pads or the amount of water sprayed until reaching 100 % of the flow when the ECT in the room is exceeded. For example, with an inside temperature of 25 to 27 °C, the cooling systems are operating, but they may turn on and off automatically at intervals. When the temperature exceeds 27 °C, they are on continually.

In geographical areas with a very high relative humidity in the environment, evaporative cooling systems are not very effective. In these cases, a **drip cooling system** may be installed to drip water on the neck of the sows when they are lying down in the farrowing crates. These systems usually alternate on and off periods. As the water on the sows' skin evaporates, they lose more body heat, which provides them with a better thermal sensation. However, their efficacy is much lower than that of the other systems mentioned.

Recommendations for drip-cooling systems

- About 330 ml of water/h/sow are required.
- The dripper flow rate should be 3-3.5 l/h.
- The recommended cycle time is 1 minute on and 10 minutes off.
- It is important to make sure the water does not drop onto the creep area.

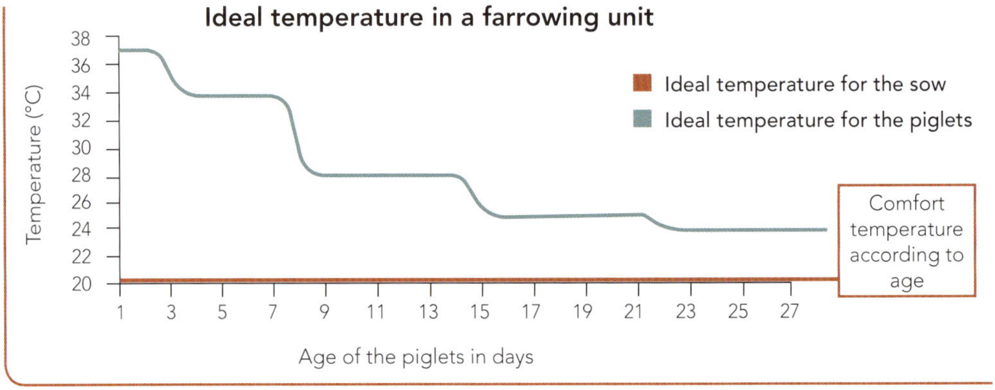

Figure 8 Temperature requirements of piglets according to their age. Adapted from Casanovas, C. *www.3tres3.com*, 2011.

Thermal comfort of the piglet

The needs of piglets for thermal comfort in the farrowing house are very different from those of their mothers, especially at birth and during the first few days of lactation. While the thermal comfort temperature range for sows is 16-20 °C, the LCT for piglets is 32-35 °C. It is therefore not possible to meet the needs of piglets only with the ambient temperature. Installing an area of extra heat for them in the farrowing pen is essential. This way, the best thermal comfort possible is achieved and the losses resulting from deaths during the birth-to-weaning period are reduced.

It is also necessary to distinguish between ambient temperature and **thermal sensation**. For example, even though the values established as temperature objectives for the sows and piglets in a room may be correct, the piglets may be seen huddled together or shivering; or they may be dispersed in the pen outside the heated area. The reason for this contradiction is that their thermal sensation is different from the real temperature. This occurs because thermal sensation is influenced by other factors in addition to temperature. These factors are described next:

- **Relative humidity of the environment**. In addition to the relative humidity of the skin, which causes latent heat losses (piglets are born wet and lose a lot of heat through their skin, which explains why they should dry off as soon as possible after birth), a high ambient relative humidity in combination with a high ambient temperature causes a greater sensation of heat and, in the case of piglets, it may favour the appearance of certain diseases. Conversely, a very low relative humidity (below 40 %) may cause dryness of the mucosae and lead to an irritating cough and a decrease in feed intake.

Table 3 Thermal sensation of piglets depending the type of flooring and air velocity. From Faccenda, 2006. In: Sanjoaquín, L. *Manejo de la cerda hiperprolífica*. Zaragoza: Servet, 2014.

Type of flooring	Outside temperature (°C)
Wet concrete slats	-10
Iron slats	-3
Concrete slats	-2
Full concrete	-1
Plastic slats	0
Sawdust	1
Straw	4
Wood shavings	5
Paper bedding	5

Air velocity	Temperature (°C)
0.2 m/s	-4
0.5 m/s	-7
1.5 m/s	-10

- **Type of flooring.** Depending on the material used, heat transmission between the body surface of the animals and the floor varies (Table 3). Plastic slats in the farrowing pens provide better comfort to the piglets than iron slats or solid concrete floors. In addition, these floors are cleaner in case of diarrhoea and facilitate cleaning and disinfection of the rooms between two litters.
- **Air velocity.** As the air velocity increases at the height of the piglets, these will feel increasingly colder (Table 3).
- **Weight at birth and vigour.** Heavier and more vigorous piglets at birth immediately start to move and drink colostrum. Their LCT decreases rapidly in comparison with the smaller and weaker piglets The farrowing house workers should provide these latter with an extra heat source and help them to ingest colostrum in order to increase their chances of survival (Fig. 9).
- **Health factors.** Piglets with early *E.coli* diarrhoea become weak, are dirty and wet and require more heat and care. Sows suffering from agalactia or mastitis also need higher temperatures.

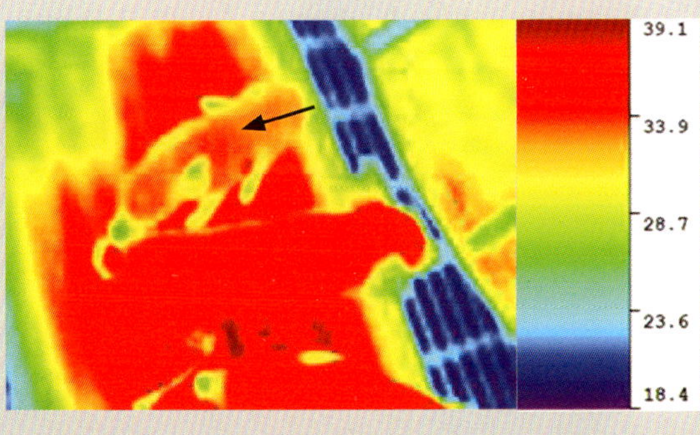

Figure 9 Newborn piglets with hypothermia (arrow) as seen with a thermographic camera. *Image courtesy of Fernando Forcada.*

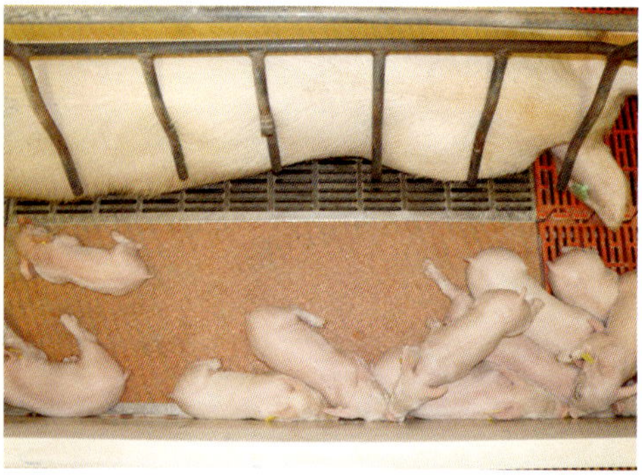

Figure 10 Piglets away from the heating pad (they are hot).

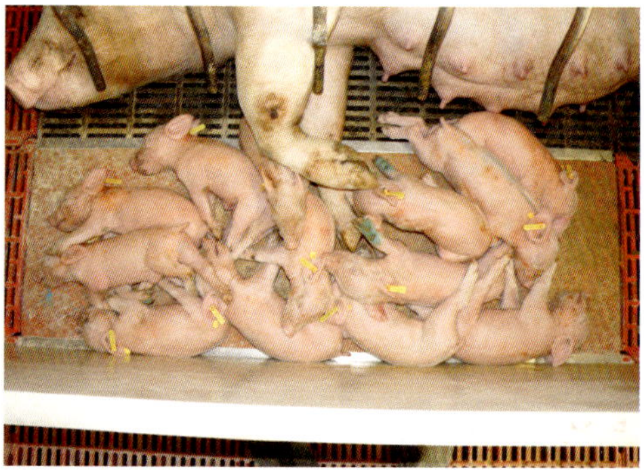

Figure 11 When the temperature is comfortable, the piglets remain on the heating pad.

All these factors affect the thermal sensation of piglets, which in turn has an influence on their behaviour. Under normal conditions, if the piglets are not suckling, they should be on the heat pads in their creep area, lying on their side. If they are huddled together or lying down on their legs, they are cold. However, if they are outside their creep area or on the border of the pads, they are likely to be too hot (Fig. 10). Under optimal conditions, the piglets should be lying down on their side and dispersed on the whole surface of the pad (Fig. 11).

To ensure the thermal comfort of the piglets, a heated area should be prepared specially for them in the farrowing pen.

Systems used to guarantee the thermal comfort of piglets

Heating pads

They are the most commonly used system on modern operations with fully slatted floors. They are made of different materials, the most common being stainless steel, plastic and polymer concrete, as they are all comfortable, hard-wearing and easy to clean. Their surface should not be rough, but it should be embossed so the piglets do not slip on it. The lower part of the heating pads should be made of an insulating material to avoid any heat losses towards the pit.

Both electric and hot-water pads are available. It is essential that the heat is distributed correctly throughout the surface of the pads so they can be used by the whole litter equally.

- **Electric heating pads.** A resistance is located under their surface and provides heat with on-off intervals. In order to function properly, they should be connected to a voltage regulator or pulse-width modulator to ensure the temperature is appropriately adjusted on their surface at all times. One regulator is usually used per room in small rooms with few farrowing pens, but the use of one regulator per row, aisle, etc. is recommended in large rooms to avoid unnecessary energy consumption. The installation of an individual switch per pad or per every two pads is also recommended so the pads can be switched on separately as the time of farrowing approaches for each sow.
- **Hot-water pads.** These pads contain hot-water pipes that transmit heat to their surface. They are connected to each other through a closed water circuit; the water comes from the boiler through a main water line, which is usually installed in the main corridor of the farrowing house. The hot water enters the rooms according to the temperature requirements for each room depending on the piglets' age.

  The system is adjusted by means of solenoid valves and temperature sensors fitted on the return pipes; all this is automated through environmental control devices.

  The disadvantage is that, due to installation costs, one single circuit is usually installed per room so that when the first sow farrows, all the heating pads in the room are turned on. In large rooms, this entails significant and unnecessary energy expenses.

  There are new pads on the market that combine an electric resistance with water; the resistance heats the water up, which then distributes the heat evenly throughout the whole surface of the pad. The initial process until the water is heated up consumes a fair amount of energy; however, these pads are very efficient afterwards, as they use very little energy to maintain the temperature.

  The **size** of the pads is also important. On highly productive operations where piglets are weaned after 21 days of age, increasingly larger pads are becoming necessary. In the past, 120 x 40 cm pads were common, which is equal to two 60 x 40 cm farrowing pads. However, on the most modern farms, the pads now installed are 120 x 50 cm if they are located in a front corner, and 150 x 40 cm if they are located in the centre or on the sides of the sow.

Heat lamps

Heat lamps are another commonly used system to guarantee the thermal comfort of piglets in the farrowing house. They consist of a lamp holder and an **infrared light bulb**, which characteristically emits less light but more short-wave infrared radiation in comparison with normal light bulbs, thereby requiring a lower filament temperature. Their power varies between 75 and 250 W and can be regulated by means of a switch in some models.

Their height can also be adjusted. They can be placed at a lower height if extra heat is required, in the case of newborn piglets for example, or elevated as the litter grows.

Heat lamps should be placed on solid surfaces (no slats), although another option would be to place a thick piece of rubber or even a water mattress, which would be more effective, below the heat lamp for the first few days.

Their main disadvantage is that their range of action is limited; in the case of large litters, only the piglets that are just below the lamp receive enough heat during the first few days. The piglets that are farther away from it may therefore be cold (Fig. 12).

To avoid these problems, the best option is to install a **covered creep area** and combine it with a heat lamp (Fig. 13). There are many different models available on the market and some handmade covered creep areas can actually work very well. They basically consist of a cover that is placed above the comfort zone for the piglets at about 50 cm from the floor. The cover should have a hole of a diameter similar to that of the heat lamp, which will be passed through the hole

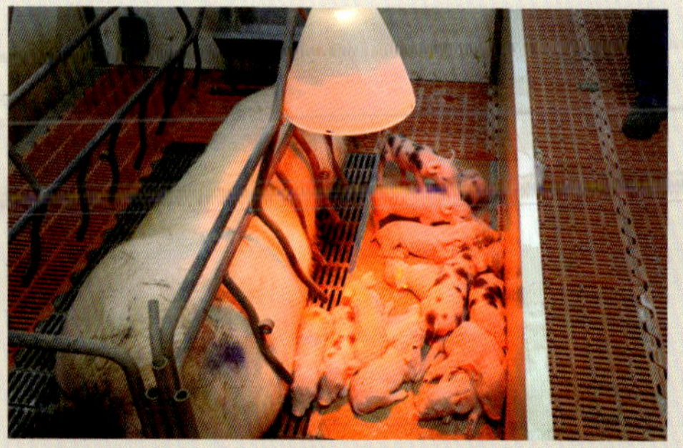

Figure 12 In large litters, the heat lamp does not provide heat to all the piglets.

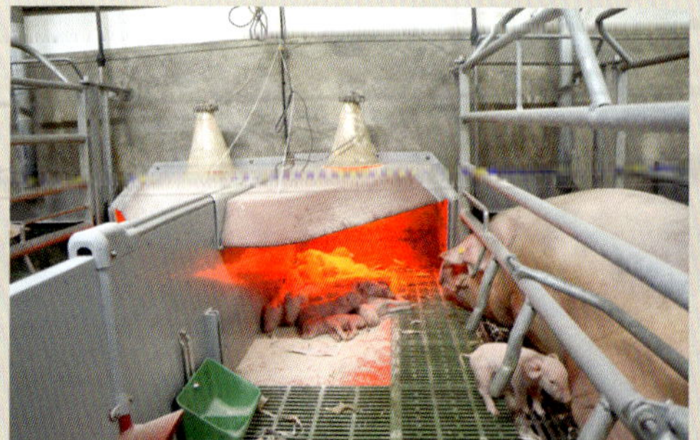

Figure 13 Covered creep area: it provides better thermal comfort to the piglets.

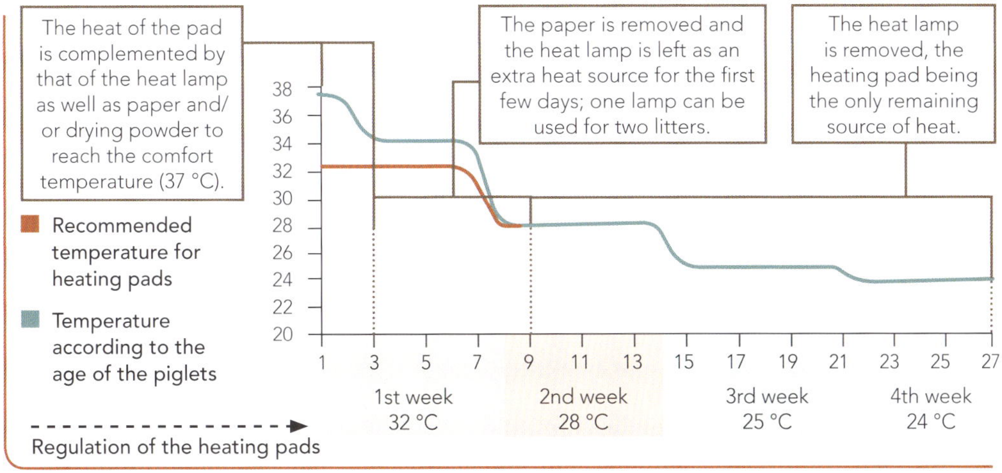

Figure 14 Combination of heating pad, heat lamp and paper to guarantee the thermal comfort of the piglets. Adapted from Casanovas, C. *www.3tres3.com* , 2011.

or anchored to the cover (Fig. 15). As the cover prevents the heat from rising, the temperature of the comfort zone is increased by up to 6-8 °C.

Covered creep areas should be well-designed and placed in an appropriate location of the farrowing pen so that management tasks are not hindered. It should be possible to lift all the covers mechanically at the same time in order to facilitate these tasks and the regular monitoring of the piglets. In the hottest months of the year, the covers should be kept lifted at all times to prevent the piglets from going to a different area of the pen with the resulting risk of crushing. Some covered creep areas allow the piglets to be kept within them, which facilitates colostrum feeding, processing tasks, etc.

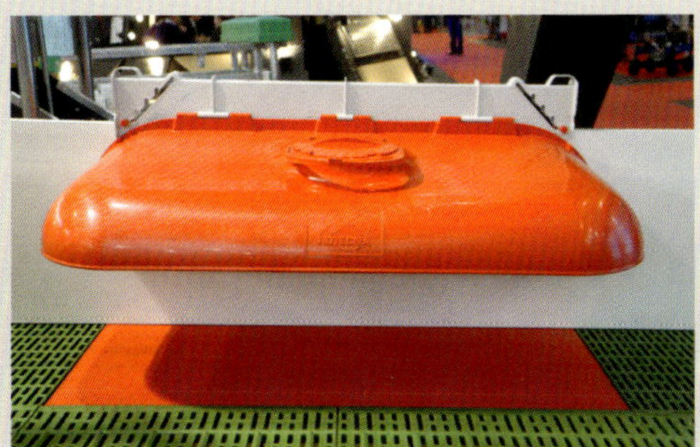

Figure 15 Lateral covered creep area. Note the opening in the cover allowing a heat lamp to be fitted.

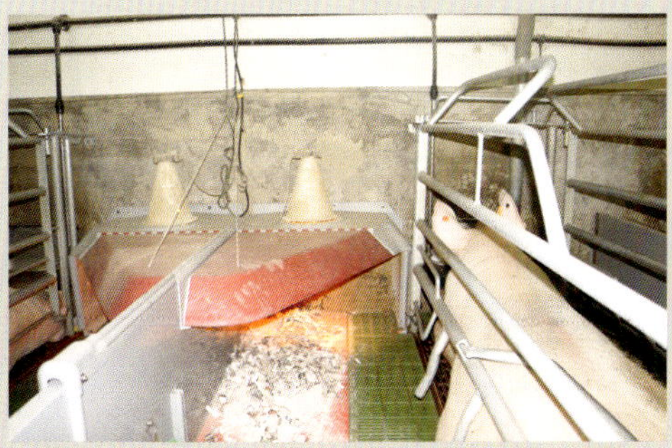

Figure 16 Ideal situation: heating pad with paper and covered creep area with heat lamp.

How can the thermal comfort of the piglets be guaranteed?

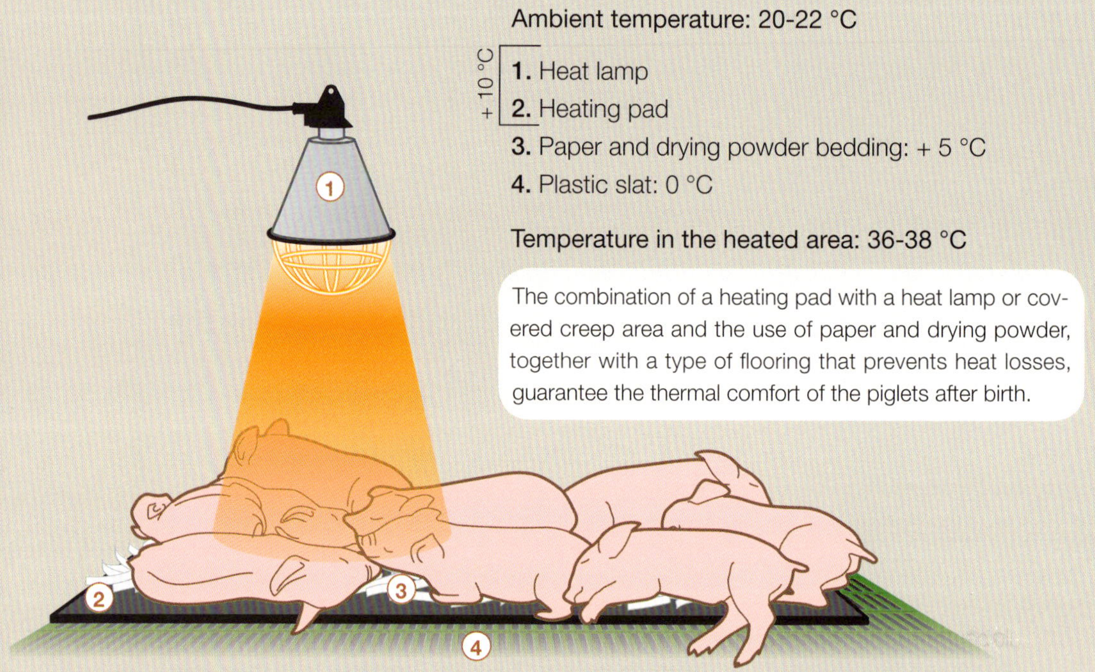

Figure 17 Ideal location of the piglets in the farrowing pen.

In conclusion, it should be emphasised that in order to produce as many piglets as possible, it is essential to prepare a thermal comfort zone and ensure it can be properly controlled so the target temperature can be modified as the piglets grow during lactation.

To minimise piglet deaths in the farrowing rooms (80% of them occur in the first two or three days), a heating pad should be used in combination with a heat lamp located above the pad (with or without a covered creep area), which will be removed on the third or fourth day of life when the piglets have overcome the most critical period. This lamp can be placed just above the rear of the sow at the time of farrowing to help the piglets dry off when they are born and avoid hyperthermia. Once the farrowing process is over, it should placed above the heated area for the piglets. Paper towels and drying powder are also highly recommended to increase the comfort of the newborn piglets (Fig. 16).

Ventilation systems

In addition to thermal comfort of the sows and piglets, appropriate air renewal must be guaranteed during the whole lactation period and at any time of the year. Ventilation systems are therefore used to provide the oxygen necessary and clean the air of dust and gases that may be toxic and harmful to both the animals and the personnel working in the rooms (ammonium, CO_2...). These systems also allow the control of ambient humidity, as excessively high values are harmful to the sow and her piglets.

Negative-pressure ventilation systems are usually used. Exhaust fans draw air from the room, which creates negative pressure and causes an inflow of outside air. These fans should be strategically placed (roof or wall) and extract air from the rooms. Outside air enters through air inlets, which should preferably be automatically adjusted and installed in the lateral walls or roof of the room, or through a perforated false ceiling (Figs. 18-20).

The fans used in farrowing houses are usually **helical and have a single-phase motor.** This allows the fan speed to be adjusted by means of digital controls that modulate tension between the terminals of the fan and make it rotate at a different speed, thereby modifying the volume of air exhausted. At low speeds, the motor is "slowed down".

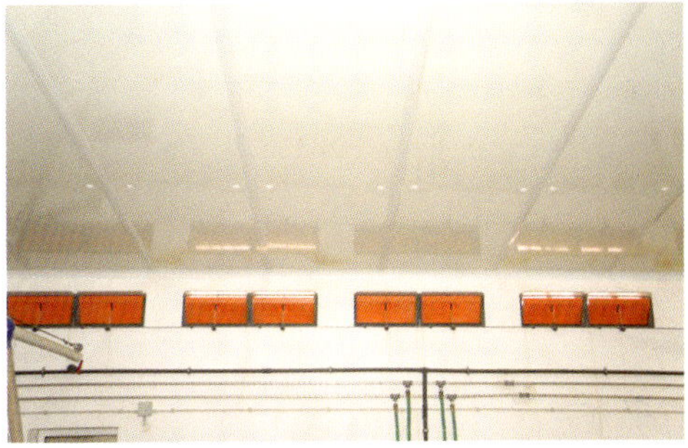

Figure 18 Air inlets in lateral wall.

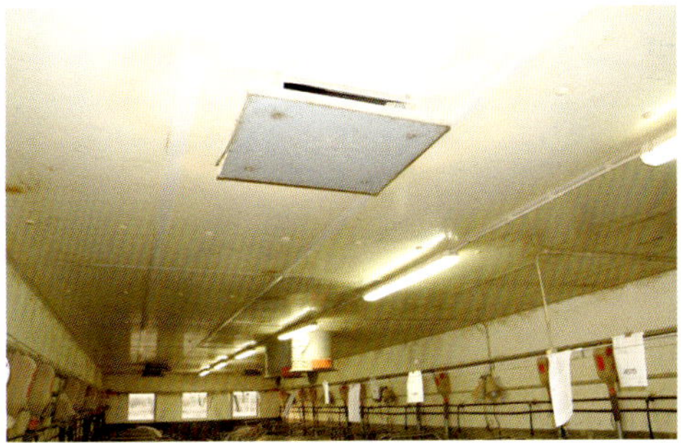

Figure 19 Air inlets in false ceiling.

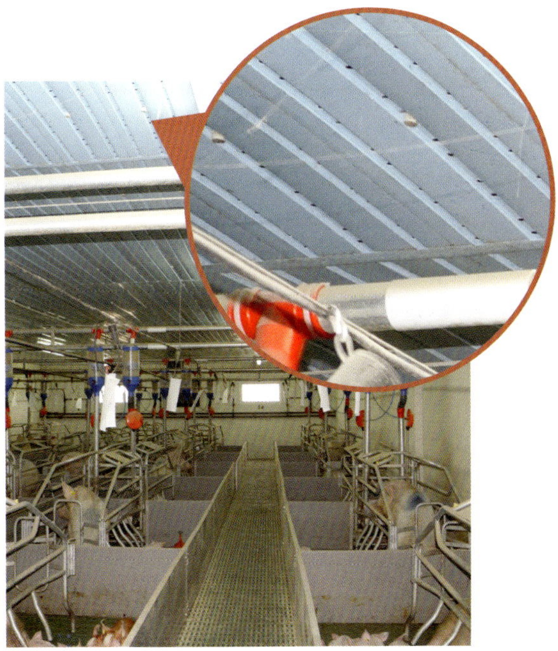

Figure 20 Perforated false ceiling.

The minimum ventilation rate (10-15 %) should be matched with a tension of at least 70-75 V to avoid overheating and enhance the efficiency and durability of the fan's motor. Single-phase motors use the same energy at low speeds as when they are working at full potential. In order to save energy (up to 40-45 %), high airflow fans with a **three-phase motor** would be recommended. Nevertheless, in small or medium-sized farrowing units, their use is not advised as it is more difficult to adjust the ventilation rate (they work in an "all or nothing" fashion) and the air velocity at the level of the animals increases, which entails some risks for the piglets.

Another option is to install **variable-frequency drives**; however, their installation is not advised due their high cost, especially in the case of small rooms. In large farrowing units, installing one per room or per every two or three rooms may be useful, provided the rooms house sows that have farrowed in the same week.

With regard to **ventilation air flows**, values of 250-300 m^3/h/sow are calculated as maximum needs (actual air flows of 180 to 250 m^3/h/sow). The number of sows in the room will determine what type of fan and how many of them should be installed.

Whenever possible, it is best to install at least two less powerful exhaust fans rather than one more powerful fan.

This way, with minimum ventilation in winter, one of the two fans will remain off, with the resulting energy savings. When the rooms are no more than 12-14 m wide, the fans are usually installed in the roof at the back of the room (an extra fan is sometimes placed in the back wall). Fresh air enters the room through the opposite wall (the wall separating the room from the main corridor); this type of ventilation is called **cross flow** ventilation. If the unit is wider, the exhaust fans should be installed in the centre of the room, with air entering through the two lateral walls. Ventilation through perforated suspended ceilings or ceilings with air inlets work well in these types of large rooms. The suspended ceiling should be installed under the roof beams to prevent the incoming air from hitting these beams and dropping directly onto the animals. In large rooms with a higher ceiling, a flat false ceiling is installed at a height of 2.4-2.5 m. This way, the volume of air to be renewed within the room is reduced, which makes air conditioning easier and contributes to significant energy savings.

It is essential to carry out smoke tests before bringing animals in for the first time, to make sure the ventilation system works correctly (Fig. 21).

Maximum and minimum ventilation rates

It is important to distinguish between the **theoretical air flow** of an exhaust fan and its **actual air flow**. The first value refers to the maximum exhaust air flow guaranteed by the manufacturer depending on the model and characteristics of the device, while the actual airflow is the maximum volume of air it can actually extract once installed.

With a negative-pressure system, the pressure difference may be affected by pressure drops at different points of the system, which in turn lead to a reduction in the maximum extraction rate. For example, when the air goes through cooling pads in summer or when the air inlets in the rooms are partially closed in winter. Therefore, these pressure drops will have to be taken into account when choosing the exhaust fans. Their maximum capacity should be equal to or higher than the theoretical ventilation requirements plus the calculated percentage of reduction in their extraction rate.

It is vital to ensure doors, windows, etc. are **airtight** to avoid unnecessary pressure drops that will reduce the efficacy of the ventilation systems. Open doors, sliding doors or simply doors that do not close tightly are commonly seen on farms where a lot money has been invested in good ventilation systems. The installation of a manometer to measure the pressure difference within the room is recommended to check that the ventilation system works correctly (Fig. 22).

If the system is well-designed, with good-quality, well-adjusted components, the maximum ventilation rates required are easy to achieve. However, the difficulty lies in maintaining a **minimum ventilation** rate to allow air renewal as well as the elimination of toxic gases, suspended particles and excess humidity, without compromising the thermal comfort of the animals, especially in the colder days of the winter season. The minimum ventilation rate is calculated as a percentage of the maximum requirements for the room and is usually about 15 %, to guarantee

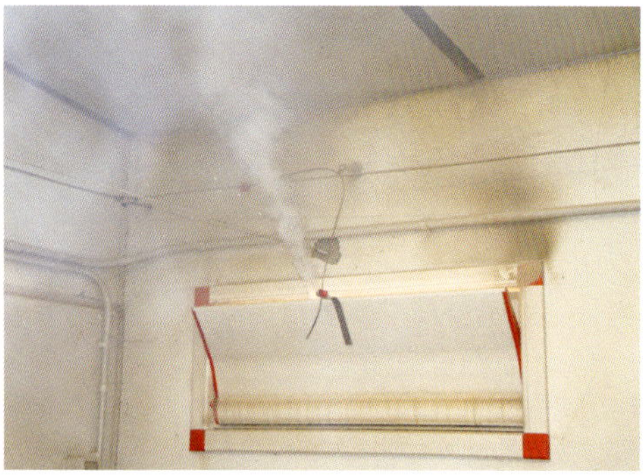

Figure 21 Smoke test in a farrowing room.

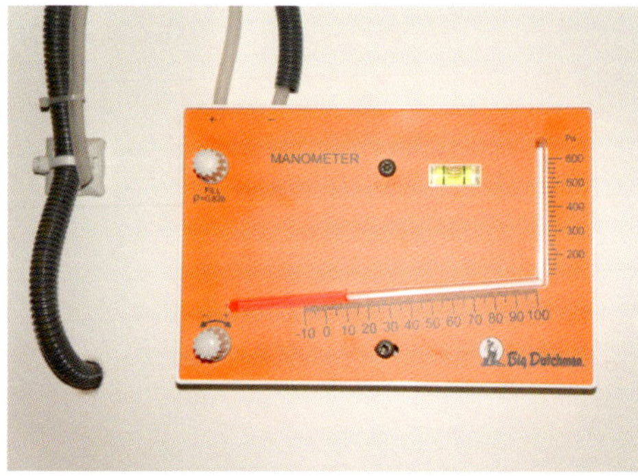

Figure 22 Manometer to control the pressure difference in the room.

sufficient air renewal and avoid unnecessary heat losses. In order for ventilation to be effective and to prevent the cold air from dropping to the piglets, the air should enter the room at a constant velocity of 1.5 m/s. In addition, cold draughts above 0.1-0.2 m/s at the height of the piglets should be avoided. This is difficult to achieve if the air inlets are controlled manually, which is why the installation of inlets with automatic adjustment are recommended.

The shutters of the exhaust fans that are not working should remain closed by means of manual or automatic systems to prevent cold air from entering in the rooms through the chimneys. The systems that work best are those in which the opening and closing of the chimney is also automatic, with a small motor and a rotary shutter (Fig. 23).

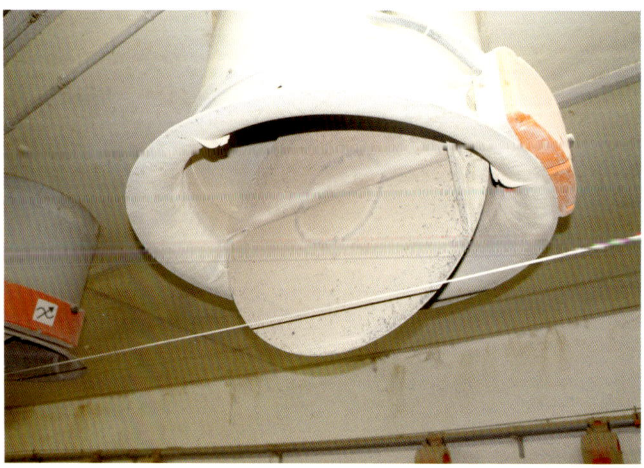

Figure 23 Automatic rotary shutter.

When there is only one exhaust fan in the room, the exhaust chimney opening should be reduced when the fan is working at low speeds.

Ventilation control

Controls

In order to ensure all the systems work properly, automated air conditioning control systems, called **controllers**, should be installed in farrowing houses (Fig. 24). These are in charge of combining the degree of opening of the air inlets with that of the exhaust fans in order to maintain the velocity of the incoming air, while cleaning and renewing the air in the rooms and ensuring the thermal comfort of the sows and, in many cases too, that of the piglets in their heated area.

They should include at least the following parameters:

- **Temperature set point.** This is the objective value that should be reached in the farrowing room. If the ambient temperature is below the temperature set point, the fans will work at the minimum set speed to provide a minimum ventilation rate. If it is above this value, the fan speed will increase according to a curve proportional to the increase in the ambient temperature, which is measured by means of a sensor installed in the room and connected to the controller.
- **Variable fan speed range.** This value corresponds to the number of degrees above the temperature set point for which the fan will rotate at maximum speed. When the temperature in the room is between the temperature set point and this temperature plus the degrees of the variable fan speed range, the fan will rotate at an intermediate speed. The higher the temperature in the room, the greater the speed at which the fans will work, but acceleration is progressive and maximum speed is reached when the ambient temperature is equal to the total temperature (temperature set point plus variable fan speed range). This reduces temperature and air velocity variations and makes them progressive, so that the animals notice them as little as possible.
  The variable fan speed range should be set between 4 and 8 °C. In situations in which there are great temperature differences (day and night, etc.), especially in winter, the set value for the variable fan speed range should preferably be increased to slow down the fan's acceleration curve.

- **Minimum and maximum ventilation rates.** The minimum ventilation rate corresponds to the minimum air flow rate required at all times to meet the vital requirements of the animals. It is usually set as a percentage (of the maximum ventilation rate). The minimum ventilation rate corresponds to 10-20 % of the maximum ventilation rate, which should be set at 100 %.

There are many models of controllers on the market, with a wide variety of functions and prices depending on the brand. The most advanced controllers offer many possibilities, such as adjusting the room temperature, ventilation, temperature of the heating pads or creep areas and turning on the cooling system when a set temperature has been reached. They also include relative humidity sensors, which turn the evaporative cooling pads or hot-pressure fogging systems off when the relative humidity in the room is above 70-75 %. The temperature and relative humidity curves of the previous 24 hours can be visualised on the controller screen to check that the systems are working properly. In addition, environmental controllers may be connected to a central computer, from which it will be possible to set the most appropriate curves for the sows in each room according to the piglets' age and time of the year. They also provide information about the temperature, relative humidity, minimum and maximum temperature parameters, etc. throughout the whole lactation, so that it is possible to make a thorough follow-up of the system's efficacy. This central computer can be accessed remotely, which allows the different parameters to be revised or changed at any time from anywhere. The installation of a camera in the rooms will enable the operation's owner or swine technicians in charge to regularly check whether the animals' comfort is appropriate.

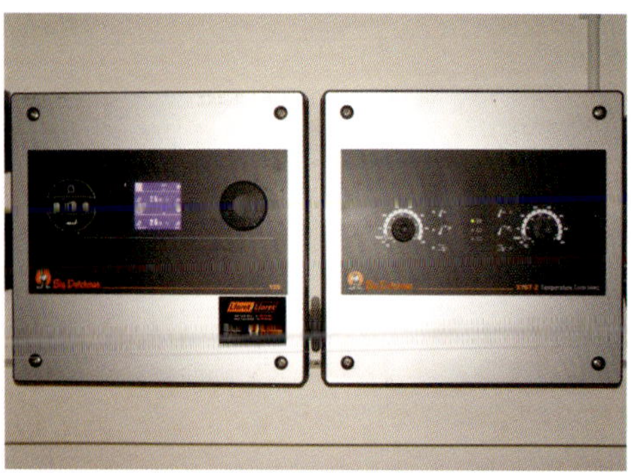

Figure 24 Controllers are devices that automatically regulate the environment of farrowing units.

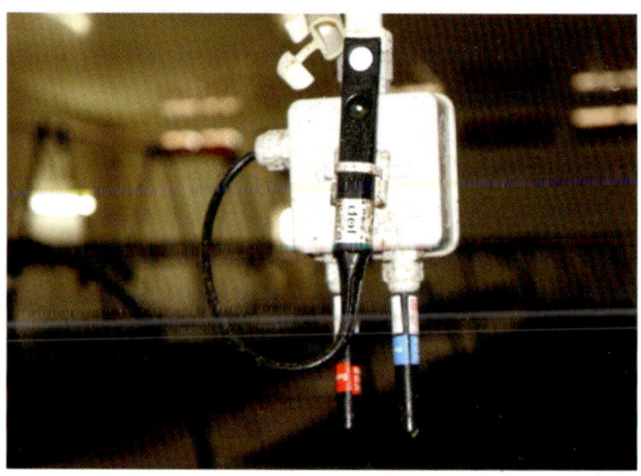

Figure 25 Triple sensor: temperature, alarm and relative humidity.

In order to reduce the cost of these systems, one controller may be installed per every two rooms, as long as the sows in each room are from the same batch (same thermal comfort and ventilation requirements). Some controllers can also adjust the parameters of two different rooms.

The installation of an **alarm system** is vital to be informed in the event of a power cut-off or if the ventilation systems stop working. Usually, these systems can send alerts to several phone numbers and activate the different auxiliary protocols (opening of the windows and air inlets, complete opening of the exhaust fans' shutters, etc.). The most modern controllers are connected to a temperature sensor with an independent alarm system in case the normal sensor fails (Fig 25). The controller notifies the error through the central computer for each separate room.

Environmental control equipment

The use of **environmental control devices** is also recommended on the farm to ensure everything works properly. These devices are economical and allow the regular inspection of the air conditioning systems on the farm, as well as the adjustment of the control parameters if necessary.

> The equipment should be thoroughly inspected every 6 months.

- **Infrared thermometer.** It is very useful to measure the temperature of the heating pads for the piglets.
- **Digital temperature and relative humidity sensor.** It can be hung in the room to compare the measurement obtained with that of the controller.
- **Anemometer.** To measure the air intake velocity and air velocity at the height of the animals.
- **Smoke bottles or kits.** They can occasionally be used as a complement to check whether air distribution is correct in the room (Fig. 21). They are usually used in newly built farrowing rooms, but regular smoke tests are recommended, as malfunctions that reduce the efficacy of the systems may appear over time and with the intensive use of the equipment.

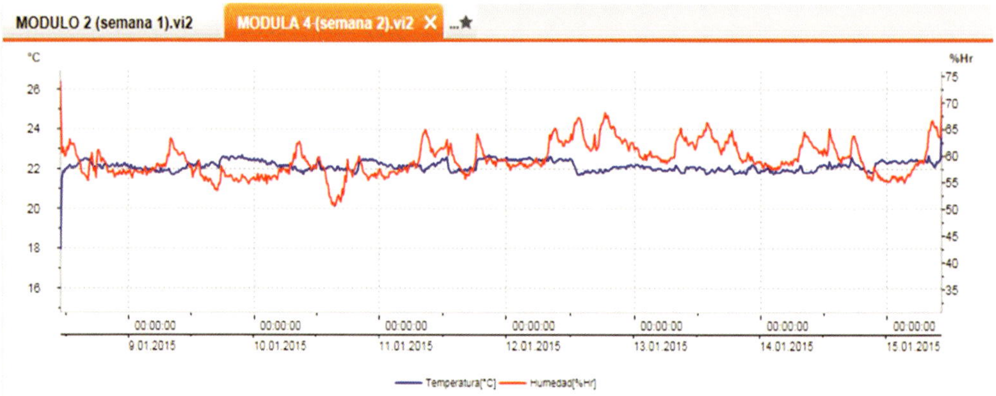

Figure 26 Example of temperature and relative humidity control graph for a room throughout the second week of lactation. *Image courtesy of Fernando Forcada.*

- **Thermographic camera.** This device can be very useful to measure the comfort of the animals. Check the body temperature of the piglets, temperature of the heating pads or heated areas, thermal bridges in the walls, heat losses at the doors or windows, etc. (Fig. 27).

The regular **maintenance and daily cleaning** of the equipment, deflectors, fans, air inlets, sensors etc. are also fundamental to achieve appropriate heating, ventilation and air conditioning in a continuous manner.

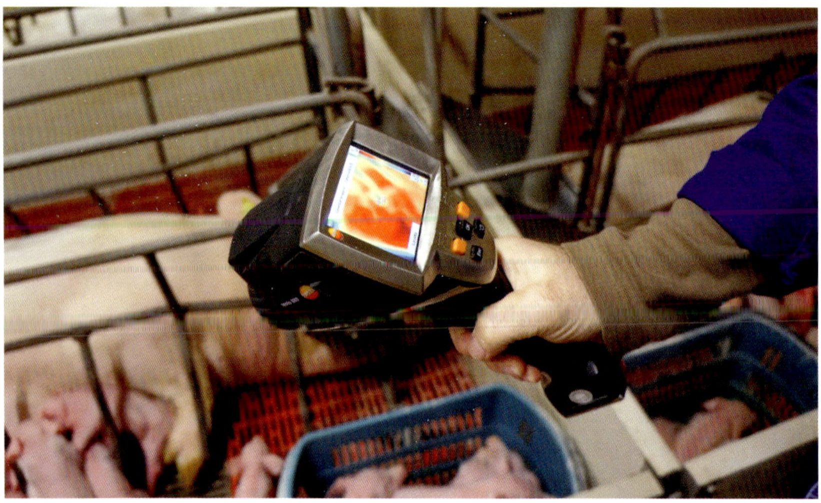

Figure 27 Thermographic camera.

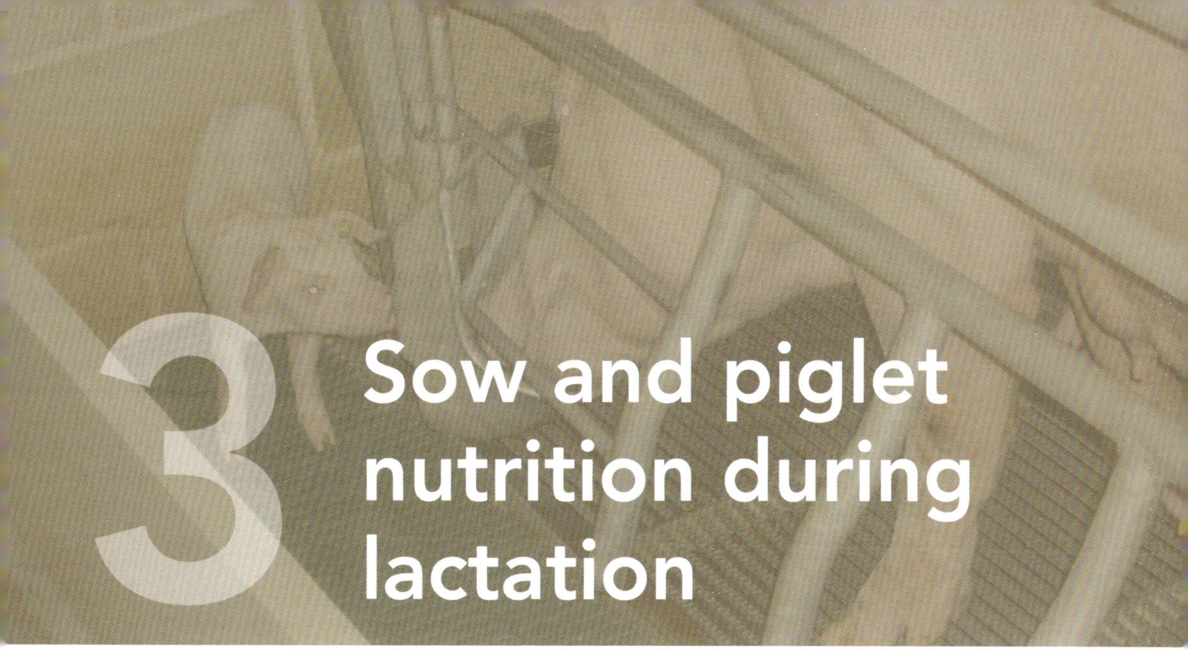

3 Sow and piglet nutrition during lactation

Basic nutrition concepts in the lactation period

The purpose of nutrition during the lactation period is to maximise litter weight at weaning, which depends on the number of weaned piglets and their weight. To achieve this objective, sows must produce as much milk as possible. Most of a sow's nutritional requirements during this period are for milk production. In addition, nowadays, sows are much leaner than 15-20 years ago and produce more milk; they also have a higher body weight in relation to their age and keep growing throughout their whole life, which results in greater maintenance requirements.

Sow feed intake often does not satisfy the requirements for milk production and maintenance and sows therefore need to mobilise their own reserves. During lactation, they lose body condition; this is observed as weight loss and a decreased amount of backfat. The latest concepts of nutrition during lactation try to minimise this loss of body condition by means of correct nutritional management during this phase.

It is considered that a sow should not lose more than 10 % of her body weight during the lactation period, and her backfat thickness should not be reduced by more than 3 mm. Greater losses compromise the following reproductive cycles by prolonging the weaning-to-service interval and by worsening future fertility and prolificacy.

Feed requirements during lactation

The sow's metabolism and nutritional requirements undergo considerable changes after farrowing. The sow shifts from an anabolic metabolic state during gestation to a state of catabolism during lactation.

From that moment on, milk production is responsible for most of the energy used by the sow (Table 1).

The amount of feed a sow needs for maintenance during lactation varies depending on her weight, as shown in Table 2.

Table 1 Energy requirements of a sow according to her physiological stage. Data provided by Martín, C. Nutrition and Formulation Service, Nanta (2014).

	Maintenance requirements (%)	Production requirements (%)
Gestation	70	30
Lactation	28	72

Table 2 Maintenance energy requirements of a sow according to her live weight. Data provided by Martín, C. Nutrition and Formulation Service, Nanta (2014).

Live weight (kg)	Maint. Req. * = 100 kcal × PV $^{0.75}$	kg feed*/day
170	4,708 kcal/day	1.62
190	5,118 kcal/day	1.76
210	5,517 kcal/day	1.90
230	5,906 kcal/day	2.04

LW: Live weight (kg)
*Maint. Req.: Energy requirements for maintenance, expressed in metabolisable energy.
**Lactation feed (2,900 kcal of metabolisable energy/kg), calculated according to NRC 2012.

The rest of the feed she ingests during this period is used for milk production. Table 3 shows the energy requirements of a sow based on her live weight and number of piglets, while Table 4 gives the protein requirements to produce milk.

The total amount of feed a lactating sow should consume is the sum of the feed required for maintenance and that required to produce milk.

From the second or third week of lactation, sows usually cannot ingest the amount of feed necessary for maintenance and for the production of all the milk their piglets need. They therefore have to draw on their body reserves. They first use up their fat reserves and draw on their protein reserves in extreme situations.

Table 3 Energy requirements of a sow for milk production in the lactation period depending on her weight and number of piglets, calculated according to the NRC 2012 with no body weight loss during this period. Data provided by Martín, C. Nutrition and Formulation Service, Nanta (2014).

		Sow (LW: 170 kg)		Sow (LW: 230 kg)	
No. of piglets	ADG g/ day litter	ME (kcal/day)	kg feed*/ day	ME (kcal/day)	kg feed*/ day
9	2,016	17,764	6.13	18,923	6.53
10	2,240	19,170	6.61	20,331	7.01
11	2,464	20,574	7.09	21,738	7.50
12	2,688	21,977	7.58	23,144	7.98
13	2,912	23,380	8.06	24,551	8.47
14	3,136	24,782	8.55	25,957	8.95

LW: Live weight; ADG: Average daily gain; ME: Metabolisable energy.
*Lactation feed (2,900 kcal metabolisable energy/kg).

Table 4 Protein requirements for production depending on milk production and weight of the sow, calculated according to the NRC (2012) with no loss of body weight. Data provided by Martín, C. Nutrition and Formulation Service, Nanta (2014).

ADG (g/day litter)	2,250		2,500		2,750		3,000	
Live weight (kg)	CP (gr/day)	SID Lys (gr/day)	CP (gr/day)	SID Lys (gr/day)	CP (gr/day)	SID Lys (gr/day)	CP (gr/day)	SID Lys (gr/day)
170	604	44	668	49	732	54	796	59
190	606	44	670	49	734	54	798	59
210	608	45	672	49	736	54	800	59
230	610	45	674	49	738	54	802	59

CP: Crude protein; SID Lys: Standardised digestible lysine.

In mid- to late lactation, a sow needs to eat more than 9 kg of feed a day in 3 meals to be able to nurse more than 12 piglets.

Water requirements

Milk is composed of 80 % water. A sow requires up to 50-60 litres of water a day during the peaks of lactation, with an average daily water intake of 30-40 litres over the whole period. A sow that does not drink enough cannot eat all the feed she requires during lactation.

In piglets, water intake is essentially achieved through milk, although water should be available for them to drink from their first day of life. During the first week of life, piglets drink an average of 50 ml a day and progressively increase their intake until reaching 150 ml at approximately 21 days of age. Once weaned, piglets need 1 litre of water a day, which corresponds to the sum of the water they drink and the water they get from milk.

The water provided should meet some minimum potability requirements (E. Magallón et al., 2014). The minimum flow should be 4-6 l/m, the recommended flow being 10 l/m. Water should be administered at mild temperatures. Extreme temperatures should be avoided as this would reduce water intake.

Drinking troughs in farrowing houses must be easy to access for the animals. Two types of drinking troughs are shown in Figures 1 and 2: a drinking bowl, which is used both by the sow and her piglets, or a specific bowl for the piglets and a different trough for the sow.

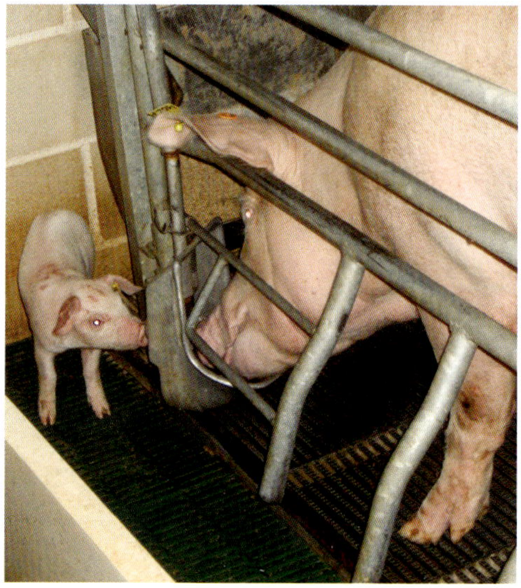

Figure 1 Drinking trough used both by the sow and the piglets.

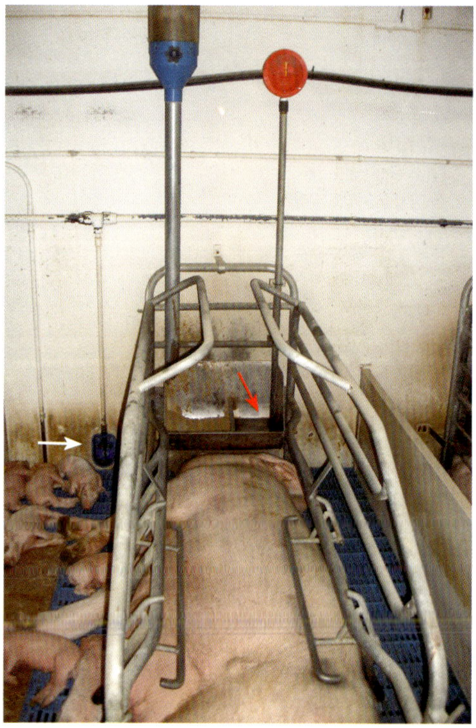

Figure 2 Separate drinking bowl for piglets (white arrow) and drinking trough with a constant water level for the sow (red arrow).

Sow nutrition

This section addresses the different factors and management systems that affect sow nutrition during lactation.

As previously explained, nutritional requirements in this phase are very high in order to prevent sows from catabolism and loss of body condition. The factors influencing nutrition during lactation are analysed next:

- **Body condition.** It has been demonstrated that if a sow gains too much weight during gestation, her appetite and, as a result, her feed intake are reduced at the start of lactation (Fig. 3). Appetite after farrowing is negatively related to feed consumption during gestation.
- **Ambient temperature.** The optimal temperature of the farrowing house for sows during lactation is 18-22 °C. For each degree above 22 °C, feed intake is reduced by approximately 100-150 g/day. This decrease can be clearly seen in Figure 4.
- **Energy and protein levels in the diet.** They should be increased in a coordinated manner, by adding lipids and amino acids. Feedstuffs excessively rich in fibre should be avoided.
- **Water intake.** Feed intake is directly proportional to water intake. The water should be potable and clean, with an appropriate flow rate.
- **Feed presentation.** Feed intake is higher with a wet diet (liquid feeding). Sows fed with liquid feed eat 10-20 % more feed than those provided with a dry diet. If a dry diet is used, pelleted feed is preferable to mash or crumbles.

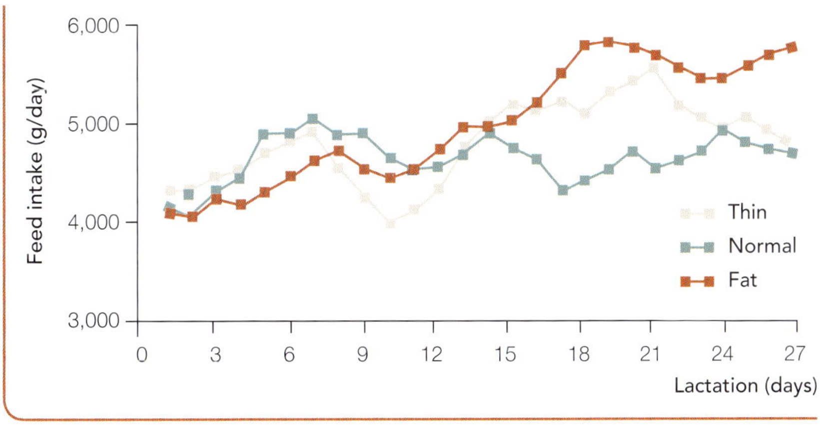

Figure 3 Feed intake during lactation according to the sow's body condition at farrowing. From Dourmad, J. Y. et al., Journées de la Recherche Porcine, INRA 1991.

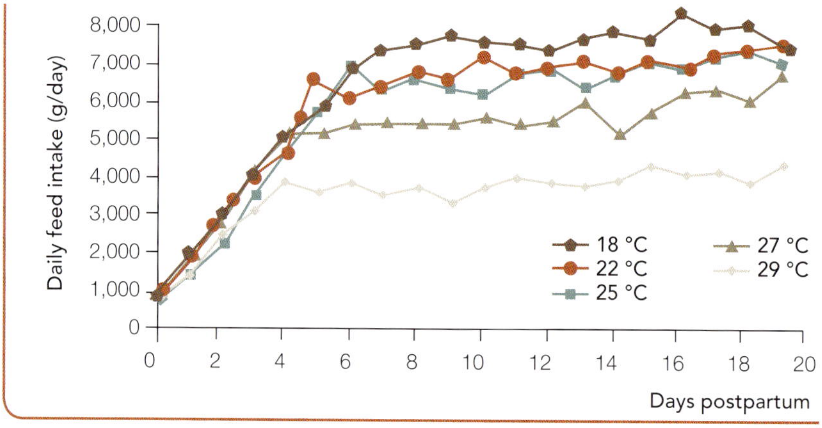

Figure 4 Feed intake of sows during lactation depending on ambient temperature. From Remaekers, P. *Nutrición de cerdas*. Nanta, 2010.

- **Hours of light.** Intake is higher with a light period of at least 16 hours a day.
- **Number and frequency of the meals.** Sows eat an average of 2.75-4 kg of feed per meal. They should be fed 2-3 times a day to increase their intake. The interval between meals should be as long as possible and sows should be fed at times of the day when temperatures are lower (sunrise, sunset...), especially in times of intense heat.
- **Number of piglets per litter and health status of the piglets.**
- **Health status of sows.** All diseases have a negative impact on feed intake.
- **Palatability.** The feed should be in good condition. It must be ensured that it is not stale, mouldy, etc. Care should be taken when formulating the feed, as ingredients with a poor palatability lead to a reduction in its intake.
- **Design of the drinking and feeding troughs.** They should be designed to ensure sows have no difficulty eating and drinking and to prevent feed and water wastage.

SOW No. ....

Lactation day	Intake				
	Meal 1	Meal 2	Meal 3	Meal 4	Total
1					
2					
3					
4					
...					
...					
...					
28					
29					
30					

Figure 5 Sample sheet to record daily feed intakes of sows in lactation.

- **Feed intake monitoring.** The amount of feed each sow has ingested should be monitored in order to give them the maximum amount they can eat without any wastage. To do so, control sheets similar to that shown in Figure 5 are used. These sheets allow workers to check the appropriate feeding curve for each sow (Fig. 9, page 56).
- **Personnel.** It is the most important factor, since farm workers are responsible for regulating and monitoring the other factors. A competent and professional workforce is essential to guarantee optimal nutritional management during lactation.
- **Facilities.** The future of feeding systems in farrowing units is heading towards individualised, electronically controlled feeding.

Feeding systems

One of the most important factors influencing sow feed intake during the lactation period is the feeding system used. The system installed on the farm should meet the following requirements:

- Automated and individualised control of the ration.
- Maximum individual intake.
- Prevents feed and water wastage.
- Reliability. The system should work under farm conditions. System failures should be minimal and easy to solve.
- Easy to clean. Feeding troughs must be easy to clean, as they should be checked daily and any remaining feed should be removed to ensure the sows eat feed in the best condition possible.

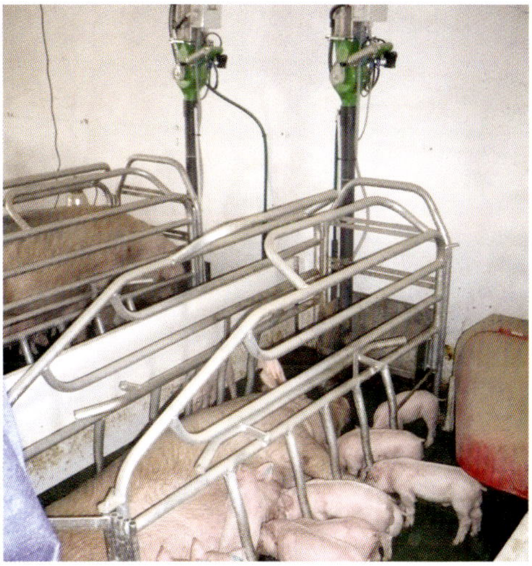

Figure 6 Liquid feeding system allowing the sow's intake to be monitored.

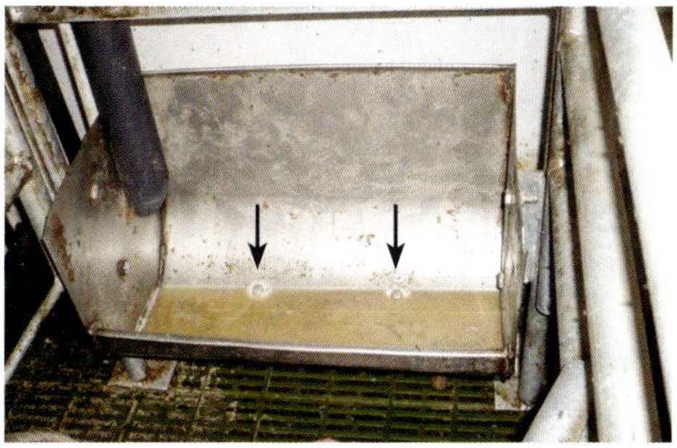

Figure 7 Detail of the liquid feeding system allowing the sow's intake to be monitored. The two sensors controlling feed and water intake can be observed (arrows).

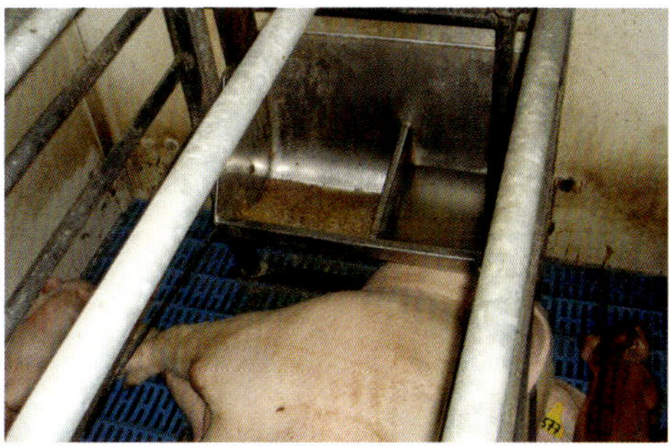

Figure 8 Trough for both dry feed and water. The water level is kept constant.

Feeding curves

Feeding curves for lactating sows should be designed by monitoring each animal's intake and adjusted to their body condition, genetics and age, as well as to the number of piglets in the litter.

Feeding curves in Figure 9 are standard curves for a multiparous sow and a gilt. A lactating sow should ingest as much feed as possible as early as possible. In the curve shown, the increment in the first week is 0.5 kg/day, with attempts to reach higher increments (0.75 kg/day or 1 kg/day). In practice, these values are difficult to achieve, especially if other factors (environment, feed, number of meals, etc.) do not help.

Designing a feeding curve involves monitoring each sow individually to keep track of her feed intake levels and adjust the feeding curve to those levels. Feed wastage should be prevented. It is thus important to control the amounts that are ingested by means of an individual record sheet, or to work with electronic systems that will show the feed intake of each sow.

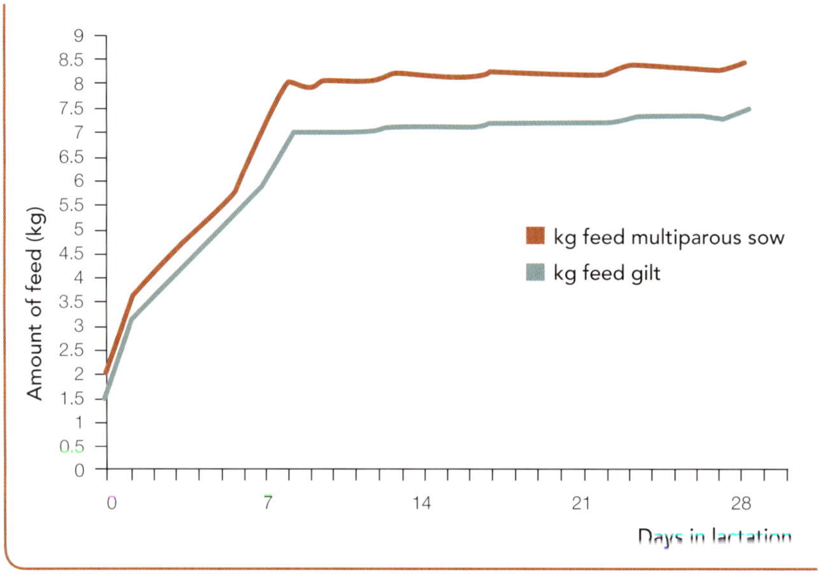

Figure 9 Standard feeding curve for a multiparous sow and a gilt (litter of eleven piglets in lactation).

Piglet nutrition during lactation

The main food for piglets during lactation is their mother's milk. Nonetheless, it does not provide all the nutrients they need to express their maximum growth potential.

The digestive system of piglets is prepared for sow's milk. However, it undergoes maturation from their first week of life, which allows them to consume special types of feed to complement sow's milk. The earlier they start eating this type of supplementary feed (solid feed), the less atrophied their intestinal villi will be at weaning.

The growth rate of piglets increases linearly from birth, while the sow's milk production decreases from the third week after farrowing (Figs. 10 and 11). When a sow does not produce enough milk or her litter is too large, two main strategies are possible: the Danish system, in which milk is provided to all the extra piglets using nurse sows, and the Dutch system, in which piglets are fed formula. In practice, both systems have advantages and disadvantages and a combination of both is often used.

Piglet growth from birth to weaning is considerable, with a weight going from 1.450 kg at birth to 6 kg when they are weaned at 21 days of age, and 8-9 kg when they are weaned at 28 days of age (Fig. 10).

It is estimated that four litres of ingested milk are transformed into one kilogram of piglet.

The use of alternative products should be assessed economically by quantifying productive benefits, the direct cost of products and the indirect cost derived from their administration (workforce, facilities...).

It should not be forgotten that the cheapest method to produce a kilogram of piglet is based on maternal milk consumption. Long lactations of approximately 28 days should therefore be favoured.

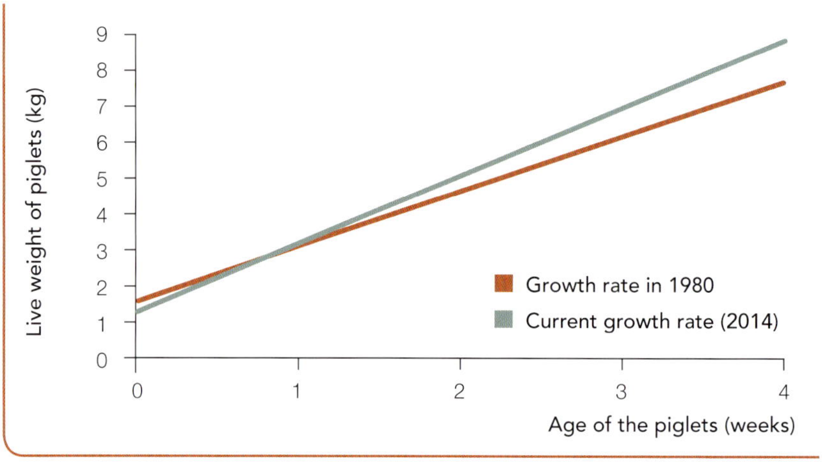

Figure 10 Evolution of the growth rate of piglets.

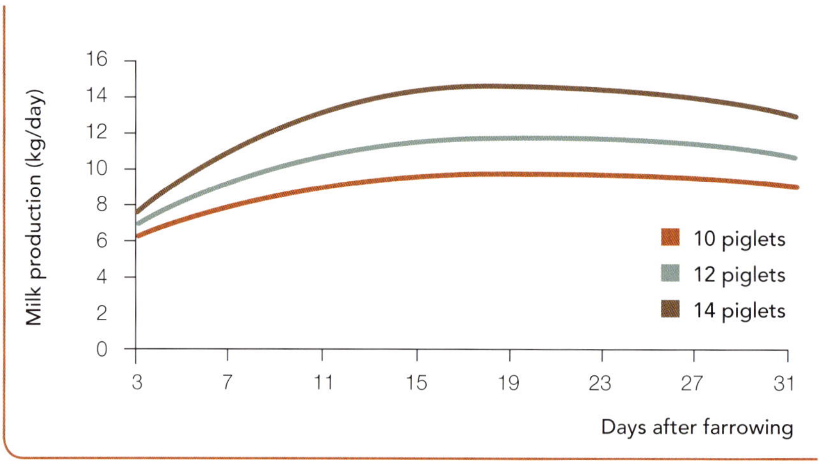

Figure 11 Evolution of sow milk production according to the number of piglets.

Formulas

They are used to feed orphaned piglets or piglets with delayed growth (e.g. from sows with mastitis), or to raise the best piglets from hyperprolific sows in productive systems in which fostering is not possible, such as with three-week batch farrowing.

Their composition is generally based on 50 % skimmed cow's milk, fat-filled whey powder, protein concentrates, vegetable fat (coconut oil), vitamins and minerals.

High-quality ingredients should be used to ensure optimal digestibility and prevent diarrhoeic disorders due to bacterial contamination or malabsorption.

Artificial nursing management to raise surplus piglets requires specific facilities: creep areas where the best piglets are placed from four days of age (Figs. 12-14). They should be provided with a very comfortable environment and the formula should be prepared in the most hygienic manner possible, bearing in mind the temperature of preparation (45 °C) and its dilution.

Formula can also be administered in pans (Fig. 15), but this method is much less efficient than management with creep areas.

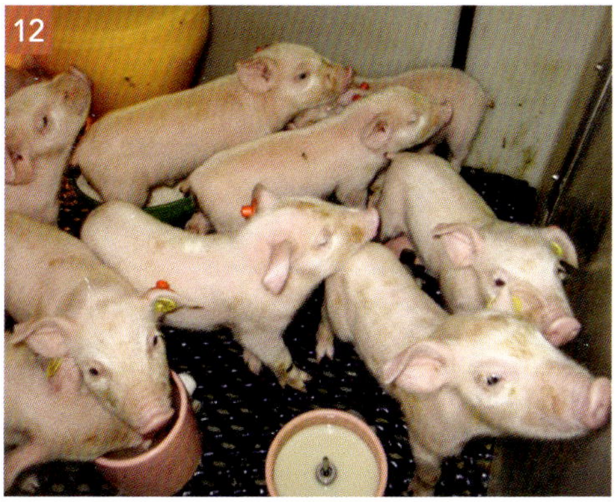

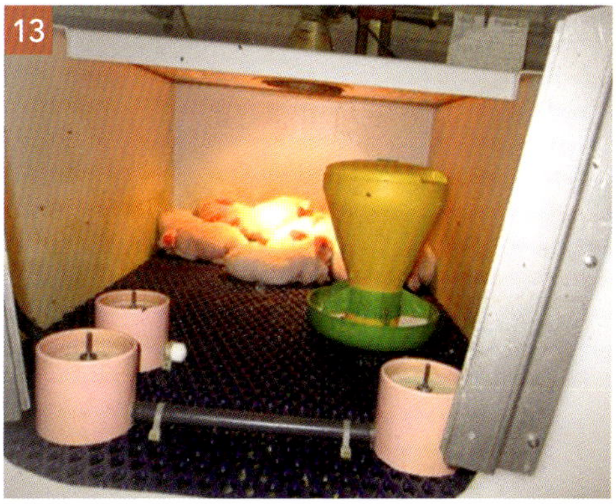

Figures 12 and 13 Surplus piglets of less than a week of age, weaned to be fed with artificial milk in creep areas. These creep areas are located above the farrowing crates.

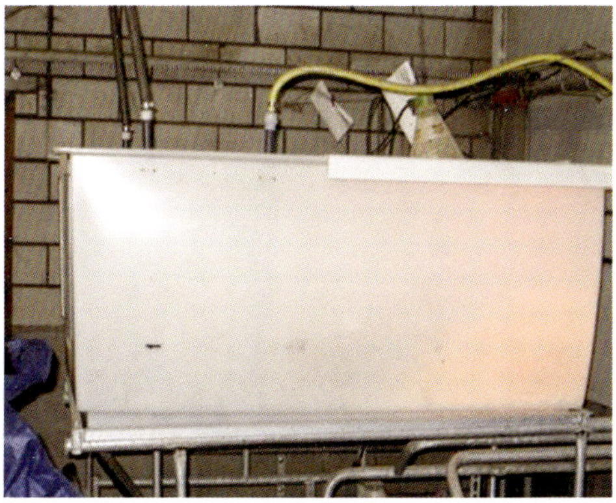

Figure 14 Detail of the location of the creep area above the farrowing crate.

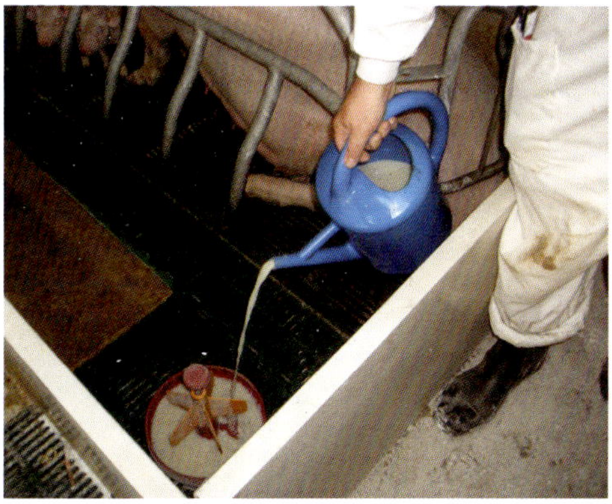

Figure 15 Administration of formula in a pan for piglets.

Creep feed

Although there are different types of feed for piglets in farrowing houses, milk replacers are usually used in the first phase of lactation, while prestarters are administered in the last third of lactation periods lasting 28 days or more.

Milk replacers are special feed formulations containing ingredients with a highly nutritive value. They are composed of whey, fish meal, high-quality soy protein, by-products of the bakery industry, flavourings, vitamins, minerals and other additives (acidifiers,...). They also contain porcine plasma. These types of feed are very rich in proteins and have a high energy value, as shown in Table 5.

Table 5 Comparison of the composition between different types of feed for piglets in lactation.

	CP (%)	ME (kcal/day)	Presentation	Recommendations of use
Milk replacer	20 %	3,500	Mash/small pellets	From 10 days of age
Prestarter	19 %	3,400	Mash/small pellets	From 20 days of age

CP: crude protein; SID Lys: metabolisable energy.

Piglets can eat milk replacers in their first week of life. However, their administration makes more sense from the second week of life (10-14 days of age).

Prestarters have similar characteristics to milk replacers. Nonetheless, as can be seen in Table 5, there are differences between the two types of feed. They should be administered from 18-20 days of age until weaning in lactation periods lasting 28 days or more. This feed is the same as that given to piglets during the first week of weaning.

Milk replacers are usually available in mash form. By contrast, although they may also come in mash form, prestarters are usually produced in small pellets of a diameter of 1.8-2.0 mm. They rarely come as crumbles.

Some farmers administer milk replacers as porridge to increase feed intake. On the first day, 1 kg is diluted into 2 litres of water and concentrations are progressively increased (1 kg of feed per litre of water). Feeding porridge is particularly recommended for small piglets.

Creep feed is administered in pan feeders for piglets, which are easily disassembled to be cleaned and disinfected (Fig. 16). Small amounts should be given with a minimum frequency of 3-4 daily meals. This type of feed is highly palatable, although the amount eaten by each piglet varies greatly (a piglet does not usually ingest more than 200 grams of feed per lactation).

It is essential to administer fresh feed in good condition. Creep feed is characterised by its flavour and palatability and should therefore be handled with care to prevent these from being altered.

Placing large amounts of feed in the pans should be avoided and the pans and feed should be kept as clean as possible (Fig. 17).

It is very important to administer creep feed to piglets in farrowing houses for a better adaptation to the weaning period.

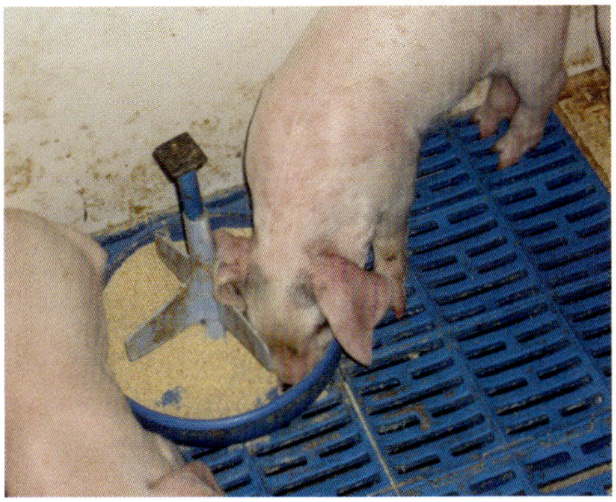

Figure 16 Pan for piglets with milk replacer.

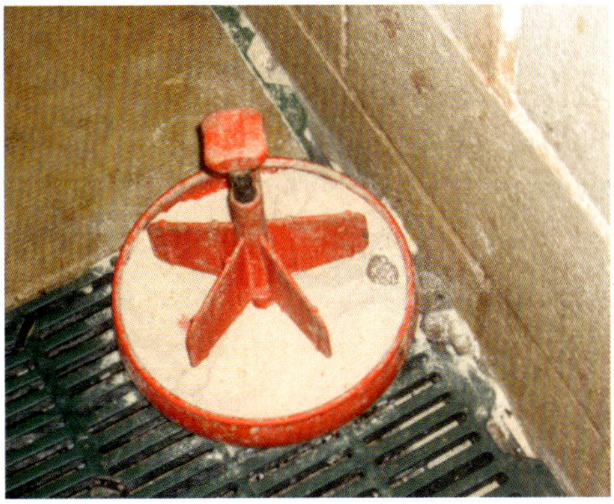

Figure 17 Pan excessively filled and dirty.

Yoghurt

Yoghurt products for piglets are actually high-energy, high-protein supplements, which are referred to as yoghurt because of their similar consistency. They are administered from the third or fourth day of life.

Their dry matter content is higher than that of milk replacers. They are prepared in a similar way to formula, but a much smaller amount of water is used.

Piglets should be fed twice daily, always ensuring the product is handled properly. The amount prepared should correspond to what piglets are going to eat at each meal so the pans are empty between meals. It is advisable to clean the pans during this interval to avoid fermentation or staling of the product.

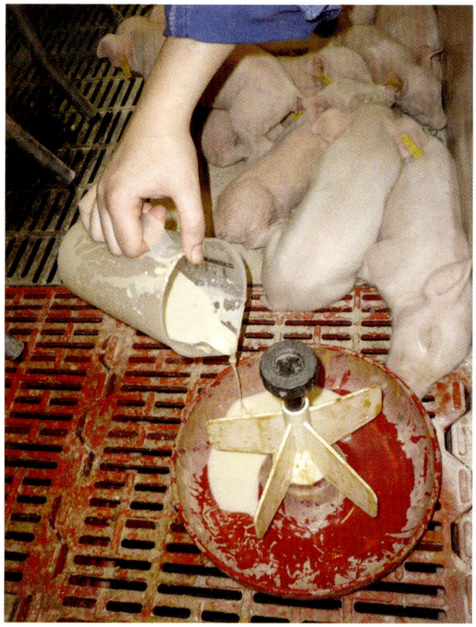

Figure 18 Pan for piglets filled with yoghurt.

Other products

Colostrum. Fresh or frozen colostrum is used for weak piglets or piglets that have not received enough colostrum during their first three days of life. Products that provide immunoglobulins essential for the immune system and nutrients that are rapidly absorbed by piglets may also be used. They are administered orally.
Gel. It is composed of energy, vitamin and mineral supplements and is administered to newborn piglets. Its composition usually includes medium-chain fatty acids, essential oils, dextrose, vitamins and minerals. With these ingredients, piglets are provided with extra energy during their first hours or days of life. The final product is referred to as gel because of its presentation in a gel-like oral paste, which is very appetising to piglets. It can be distributed in pans or administered directly in their mouth by means of an applicator.
Others. Prebiotics, vitamin complements, algae...

In the past few years, given the large numbers of piglets produced, a variety of nutritional supplements have appeared to try to make up for the insufficient amount of milk produced by sows. Their efficacy is questionable and they are only useful for excess piglets on farms with systematic digestive disorders.

Systems to monitor feeding levels on the farm

Given their importance, feeding protocols should be clear and simple. Any member of the personnel working on the farm should know and understand them.

Sow feeding at any productive phase –especially during lactation– should be controlled individually taking into account the animal's body condition and physiological stage.

On operations with electronic feeding systems, a programme sets the curve for each type of sow after adjustment of the different parameters by the farm personnel. The programme includes a series of predefined curves and the person in charge then decides which is the most appropriate for each animal. The body condition of sows should be checked weekly to adjust their feeding curve.

Sows on operations without automated feeding systems should be monitored daily, and their feed dispensers should be adjusted based on their body condition and the variations in the density of the feed.

In both cases, the protocols should include:

1. Individual monitoring and/or recording of the sows' body condition.
2. Grouping the sows that are at the same physiological stage based on their body condition.
3. Adjusting the dispensers based on the feeding curves chosen according to the animals' body condition.

Several methods can be used in order to monitor body condition (Table 6). It is essential to use one or several of them on a routine or systematic basis.

Table 6 Comparison of the different systems for body condition monitoring. Adapted from Collell, M. *Alimentación de la cerda en gestación*, 2007.

	Visual control	Body condition scoring	Weight	Ultrasonic measurement (backfat thickness)	Measurement with a measuring tape
Time necessary	+	++	++++++	+++	++
Accuracy	+	++	+++++	++++	+++

Visual monitoring

Determining whether a sow is thin or fat with the naked eye is a fast but subjective method, as there are no precise and clear references. Visual monitoring should always be performed by the same person and complemented by other methods.

Body condition scoring

It is a very typical and frequently mentioned method. The ideal body condition corresponds to a score of 3. Very thin sows (body condition score = 1) will never be able to express their full productive potential, and very fat sows (body condition score = 5) represent an unacceptable extra economic cost for an operation, in addition to having severe reproductive problems (dystocia) and a very low milk production.

Monitoring feeding levels based on body condition is a rather subjective method. For this reason, it should preferably always be done by the same person. This method is somewhat inaccurate but it is used on a routine basis as it is easy to apply as part of the different tasks to perform on the farm (Table 7 and Figs. 11 to 23).

Table 7 Gestating sow feeding. Correction of the ration according to the sow's body condition. Adapted from Martín, C. Master2Know, 2012.

Feeding programme according to body condition.					
Body condition	1	2	3	4	5
	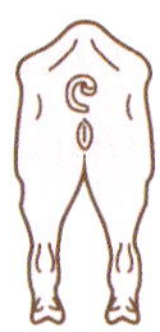	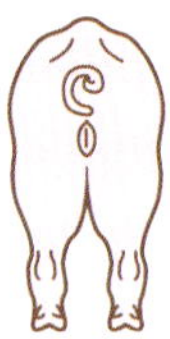	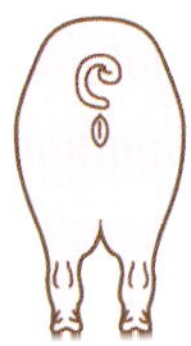	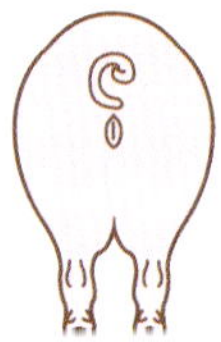	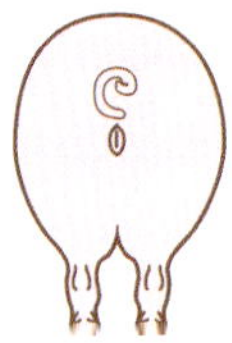
When should the sow be in this condition?	Never	Weaned	Beginning of gestation	End of gestation	Never
Are the bones of the spine and pelvis visible?	To the naked eye	With slight pressure of the hand	Felt when pressing firmly with the hand	They cannot be felt when pressing with the hand	Overall aspect: very fat
Correction of the base ration (kg/day)	+0.6	+0.3	Correct	-0.3	-0.6

BODY CONDITION OF SOWS UPON ARRIVAL AT THE FARROWING UNIT

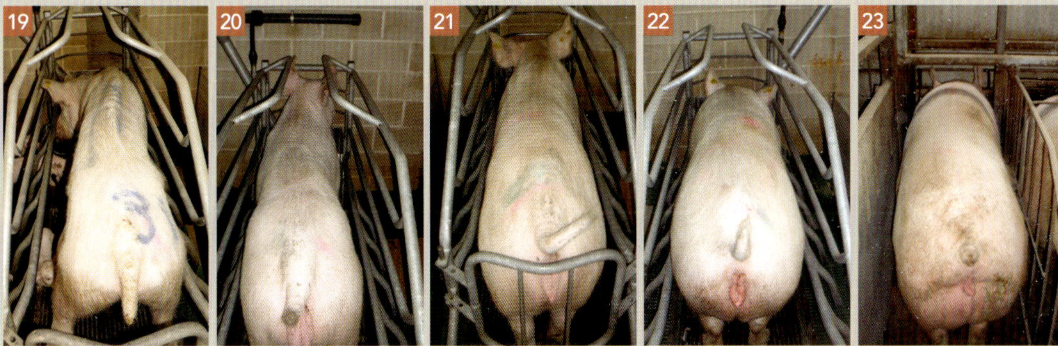

BODY CONDITION 1	BODY CONDITION 2	BODY CONDITION 3	BODY CONDITION 4	BODY CONDITION 5
Very thin	**Thin**	**Optimal**	**Fat**	**Very fat**

Individual weight monitoring

Very objective and precise method. Not very practical under current farm conditions; mainly used in experimental studies. It will surely become useful in the near future, as new technologies will make it possible to install weight scales in the aisles, pens and in electronic feeding stations.

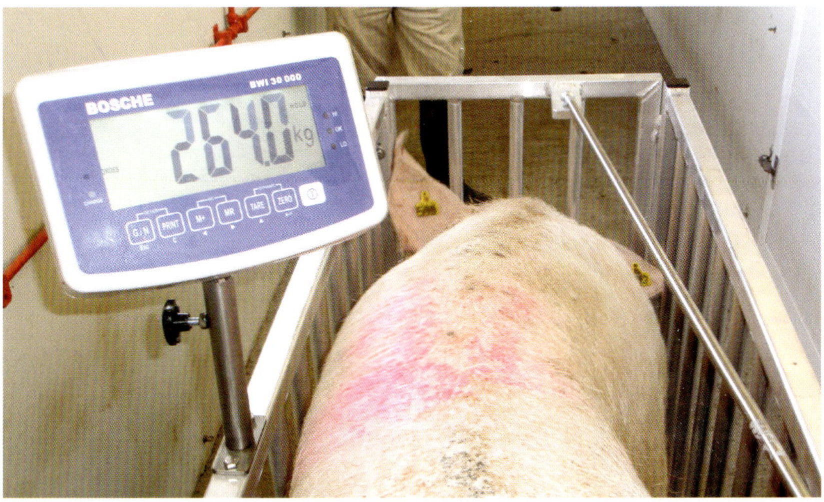

Figure 24 Individual weighing of gestating sows upon arrival at the farrowing unit. *Image courtesy of José Manuel Mancera.*

Backfat monitoring (P2)

Backfat thickness is measured by means of an ultrasonic instrument, which consists of a probe and a display unit showing backfat thickness in mm (Table 8, Fig. 25).

Table 8 Recommended backfat thickness (P2), based on the age and productive stage of the sow (for lean sows with a body condition score of 3). Recommendations from the authors, 2014.

	Backfat thickness		
	Service	Farrowing	Weaning
Multiparous sows	13-15 mm	16-18 mm	13-15 mm
Gilts	14-16 mm	16-18 mm	13-15 mm

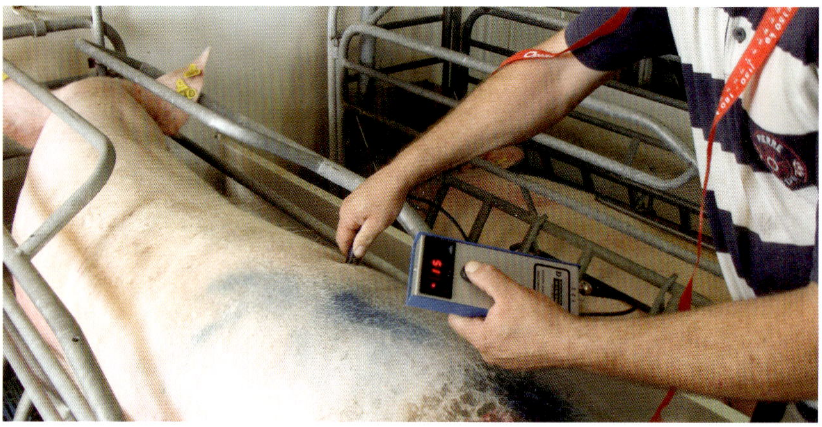

Figure 25 Measurement of backfat thickness at P2 using an ultrasonic device.

Procedure

When using this device, the probe must always be placed at the same point, at the level of the last rib, 65 mm from the median line (this is referred to as the P2 point) (Fig. 26).

Areas with a large amount of hair should be avoided. If necessary, the area should be clipped of hair and ultrasound gel –or failing that, oil– should be applied on the probe, as no air should remain between the probe and the sow's skin. This method is sometimes inaccurate as differences are observed in the measurements obtained depending on who performs the procedure and where the probe is placed.

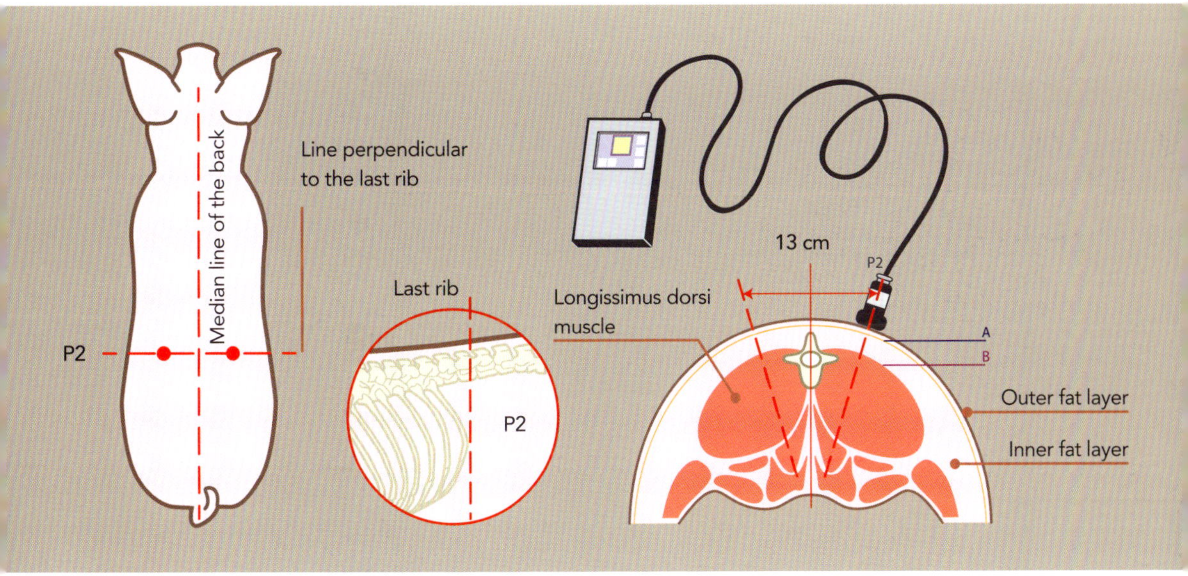

Figure 26 Location of the P2 point (65 mm from the median line, at the level of the last rib) to measure backfat thickness. A: Separation of the fat layers. B: Fat-muscle limit.

Backfat thickness can also be measured by means of ultrasound imaging devices. Linear transducers are normally used, as they provide an image from the first millimetre in contact with the skin, which allows great measurement accuracy. Sector transducers are also suitable for backfat thickness measurement; the image they provide is less clear but they are much easier to use. They are used in a similar way to ultrasonic probes and the measurements are taken at the same point of the animal.

> Increasingly leaner sows are selected, as this has a positive influence on their offspring's feed conversion rates.

It is important to monitor sows according to their age and physiological stage in order to be able to see and study their evolution.

Their genetics should be taken into account. Nowadays, the new lines are very lean, and backfat thickness values that years ago used to be a reason for concern are now considered normal. Sows will probably be even leaner in the future.

Weight monitoring using a measuring tape

This method involves measuring the sow with a measuring tape specific for this purpose, which relates the distance between the sow's two flanks with her weight. Measuring this distance provides an approximate weight for the sow.

This procedure is more laborious than visual body condition monitoring, but it is more objective and more accurate values are therefore obtained. Accuracy will depend on the genetics, physiological stage and cycle of the sow.

In practice, it is recommended to monitor the sows' weight weekly with one method –including at least body condition scoring– and to adjust their ration according to their body condition. For greater accuracy, the best option is to use body condition scoring along with backfat measurement or measurement using a measuring tape. The most objective and accurate method is individual weighing in order to evaluate the sow's weight on arrival at the farrowing house and at weaning and to determine the degree of body condition loss and most appropriate nutrition levels.

With these measurements, any deviations in a sow's body condition can be corrected and nutrition levels adjusted.

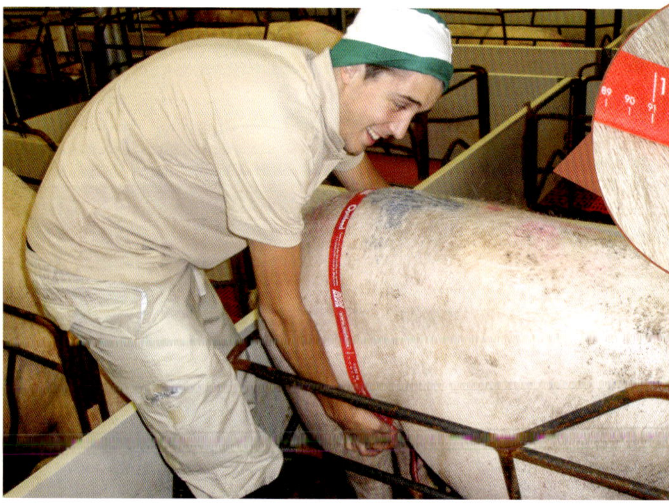

Figure 27 Weight measurement with a measuring tape in a farrowing unit. *Image courtesy of José Manuel Mancera.*

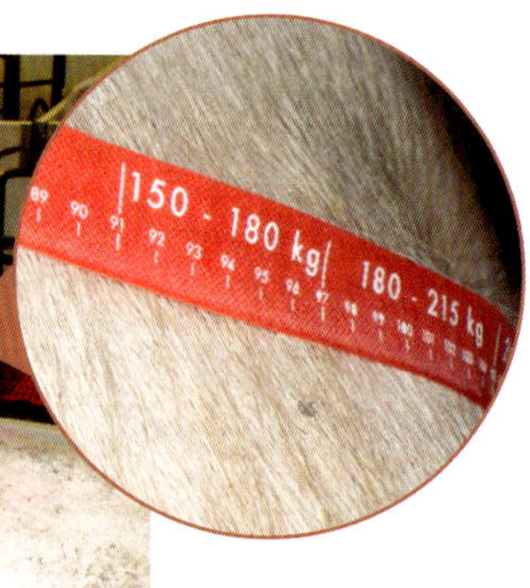

Figure 28 Detail of the measuring tape used, on which the correspondence between weight and distance in centimetres can be observed.

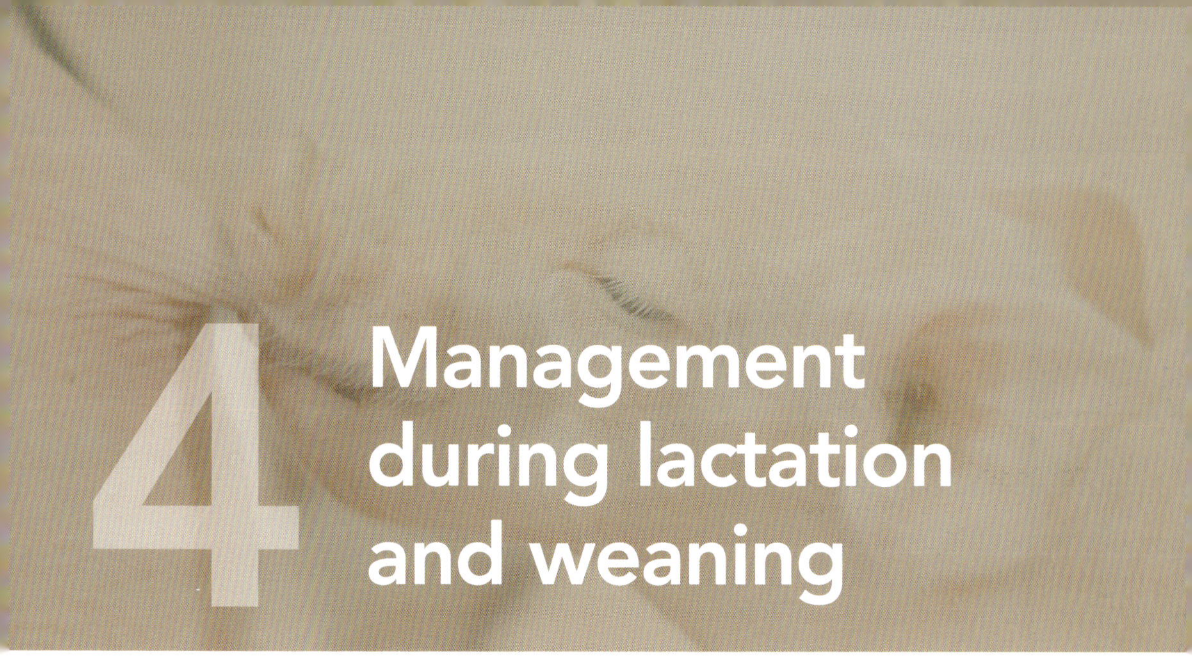

4 Management during lactation and weaning

Introduction

Hyperprolific sows usually farrow more piglets than they can nurse; this is one of the main problems to be solved in modern swine production.

Many piglets are small and lightweight at birth, and sows are unable to produce enough milk to nurse all the piglets born alive. Moreover, as they become older (more than 5-6 farrowings), their milk production capacity decreases and some of their teats become non-functional due to lesions, mastitis, etc.

The genetic improvement responsible for sows' enhanced prolificacy has taken place faster than the genetic improvement in terms of increase in the number of teats and milk production capacity. It is therefore common to have sows with more piglets than functional teats.

It is very difficult to get a sow with 14-16 live born piglets to nurse all of them by herself.

This chapter reviews the different strategies to solve this problem.

Management during lactation

This section will only refer to the system in which sows are housed in farrowing crates. They can also be kept in loose housing from the very day of farrowing or from the fifth day of lactation, but this practice is very uncommon on commercial operations. This system is used almost exclusively in experimental settings in research centres to study animal welfare or behaviour, as well as in some Northern European countries.

Environment in the farrowing unit

Maternal instinct is decisive when it comes to establishing the mother-offspring bond and achieving a good start to lactation. The farrowing unit must have a perfect environmental control that provides a state of comfort to the sows and prevents them from getting nervous, so they can concentrate on milk production and on nursing their piglets.

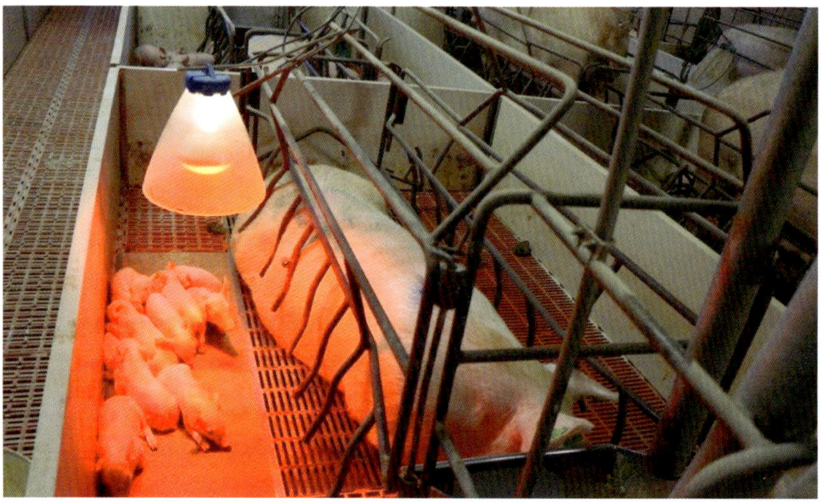

Figure 1 Farrowing room with a quiet environment.

Postpartum management

Piglet management

At 12-24 hours postpartum and after ensuring the piglets have ingested sufficient colostrum from their mother –either in a natural manner or by means of techniques such as split suckling– the litters are evened out in number and size in each farrowing room. The sows' prolificacy and number of functional mammary

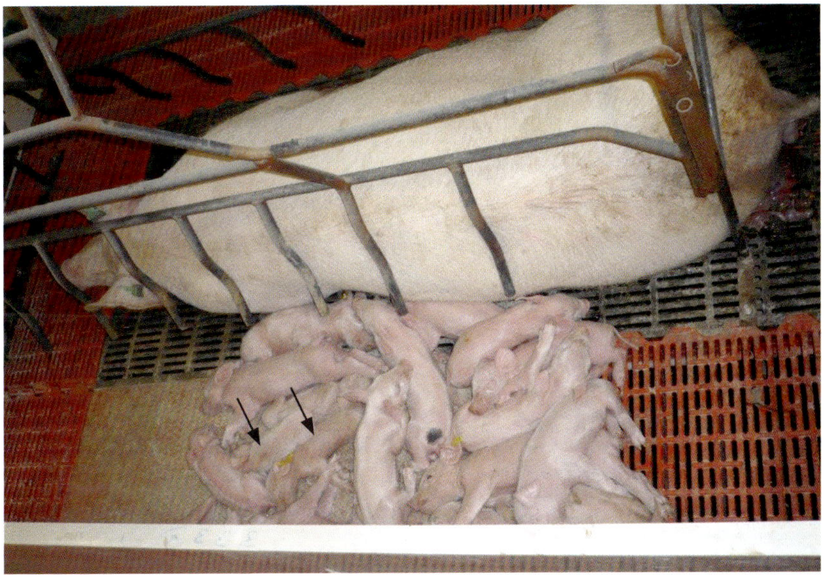

Figure 2 Large litter with some runt piglets (arrows).

glands should always be taken into account, as well as the shape and size of their teats, so the piglets are placed with sows according to the teat morphology of these latter.

Once the piglets have been placed with sows in a homogeneous manner, they should not be moved again. As seen in previous chapters, pigs are very hierarchical animals; fights for the best teats take place from the very first day and piglets will always nurse from the same teat from their second day of life.

Piglets should preferably be processed at three days of age, when they are more vigorous. It should be remembered that more than 80 % of the deaths occurring in the birth-to-weaning period take place in the first three days of life. In addition, the small injuries caused to piglets when they are processed (tail docking, vaccines, iron administration, ear-tagging) are a cause of stress and lead to an increase in mortality, especially in weaker and smaller piglets.

More than 80 % of the deaths occurring in the birth-to-weaning period take place in the first three days of life.

Gilt management

Gilts are given as many of the largest piglets as possible, 12 to 14 minimum, depending on the farm's productive performance levels and on the genetic line. The purpose is to activate as many teats as possible so these sows have a good mammary development for the rest of their productive life.

It is crucial that gilts reach farrowing with a good body condition thanks to a good diet and appropriate age at first service. This latter parameter will vary according to the different genotypes and nutritional strategies. In general, a minimum of 7-8 months of age and 140 kg of live weight are recommended. Gilts should have also come in heat twice before their first service.

Figure 3 Behaviour of the nursing piglet. Adapted from Quiles, A. and Hevia, M.L. *Cría y Manejo del lechón.* Ed. Acalanthis Comunicación y estrategias, 2006.

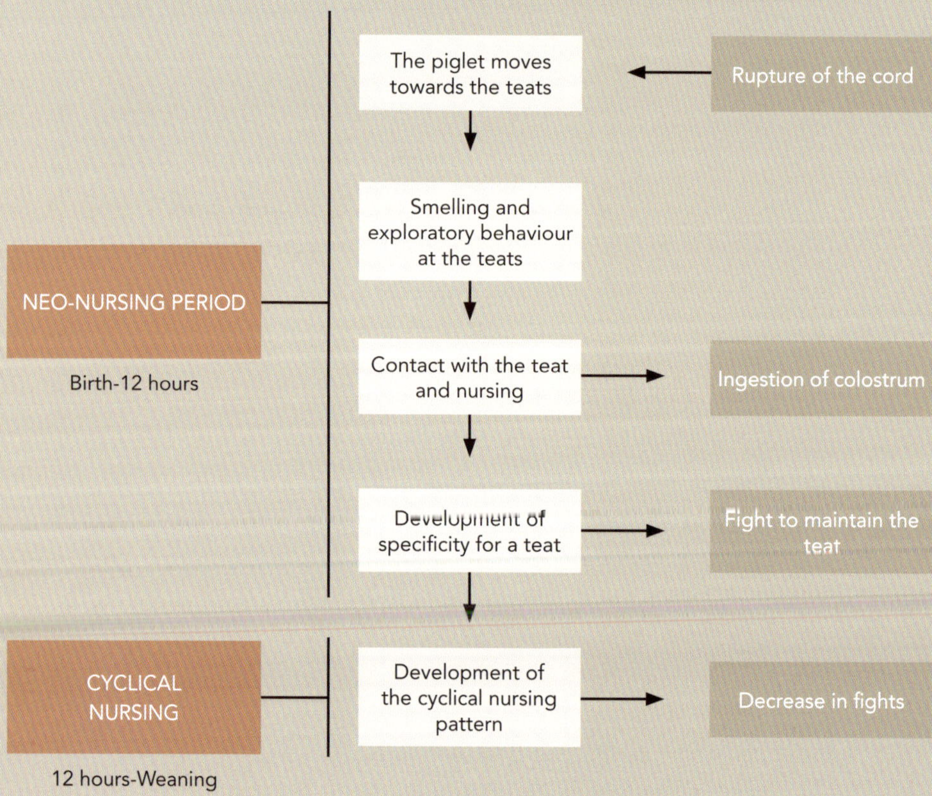

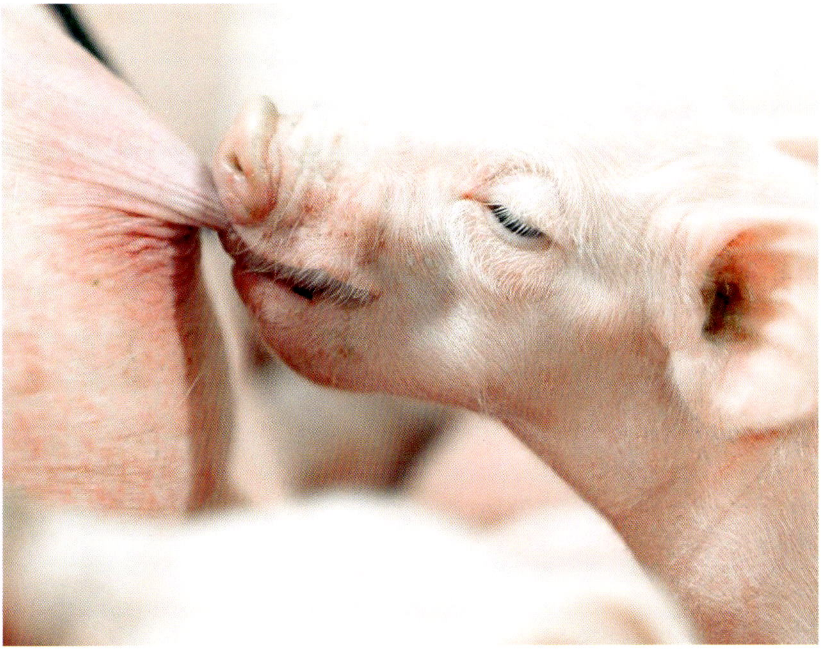

Figure 4 Newborn piglet nursing. *Image courtesy of Nutreco.*

Management practices during lactation

Lactation rapidly goes from **neo-nursing**, which corresponds to the first day after farrowing when colostrum is available to piglets at all times, to **nursing cycles** with each piglet nursing from the same teat every 40-60 minutes.

Surplus piglets are placed with nurse sows (see Chapter 6) or given supplementary feed. Both strategies are often combined.

Sows should be in perfect condition at the start of lactation and it is therefore essential for them to have access to sufficient water and feed.

> It essential for sows to have access to sufficient water and feed so they are in perfect condition at the start of lactation.

Management strategies during lactation

When faced with the challenge of a hyperprolific sow with more piglets than teats that cannot nurse all her offspring, swine farmers establish different strategies:

- **Based on providing more natural milk to the piglets**: mainly through feeding programmes adapted to this phase and aimed at maximising the sow's feed intake to favour a good milk production, or through techniques that prolong the lactation period of some sows, such as the use of nurse sows or group suckling.
- **Based on providing the piglets with supplementary feed**: milk replacers, yoghurt, gels, nutritional supplements... at increasingly earlier ages or by means of artificial lactations. These are achieved by weaning piglets at very early ages and feeding them formula in special creep areas or, on occasions, by weaning the strongest piglets in a litter a week before the usual time of weaning for the operation.

In practice, a combination of several of these strategies, which are described next, is used in most cases.

Increasing the amount of natural milk available to piglets

This is mainly achieved with nurse sows, but also with other techniques that are no longer used on a frequent basis such as group suckling and intermittent suckling. These techniques are explained next because of their experimental interest.

Cross-fostering

This is the most common system used on the most modern operations with hyperprolific lines throughout the world. The cross-fostering or Danish system is explained into greater detail in Chapter 6.

In essence, it lies in making young sows –mainly those that have farrowed twice or three times– have two consecutive lactations: they will nurse their litter and then a second litter, thereby prolonging their lactation.

Cross-fostering is possible thanks to the extraordinary milk production capacity of sows, which results from their capacity to convert feed into milk. It is therefore essential to feed them appropriately in the farrowing unit.

Group suckling

Until a few years ago, it was quite common, from the piglets' second week of life, to see farmers opening the lateral partitions of the farrowing pens to facilitate group suckling and allow the piglets from two, three, four or even six different litters to nurse from one sow or another indistinctively.

This was done in order to help the weakest litters or as a result of an insufficient milk production by some of the sows. This practice is no longer advised nowadays, as it has more disadvantages than advantages: it does not solve the insufficient milk production of some sows caused by mastitis or other problems, and the strongest piglets nurse more, which gives them an even greater advantage over the smallest ones. The only advantage is that it facilitates the socialisation of piglets from different litters.

The alternative to this technique is to treat any problematic sows and, if necessary, to move the litter to another sow or wean the piglets early using alternative feeding: milk replacers, yoghurt, formula, etc.

Intermittent suckling

Intermittent suckling involves separating the sow from all her piglets in the days prior to weaning (2 to 12 days) for a variable period of time (between 2 and 12 hours), during which they are administered feed. The objective is to favour the physiological adaptation of the piglets to weaning, a phase in which they will change from a highly digestible liquid diet (milk) to a solid and less digestible diet (feed). This technique favours their feed intake and adaptation to the post-weaning period. It has been demonstrated that when piglets eat feed during the lactation period, even in very small amounts, they adapt better to the weaning process since their digestive system is better prepared for feed consumption.

This management technique is used almost exclusively at experimental level and may be of interest in the future.

It has been demonstrated that when piglets eat feed during lactation, even in small amounts, they adapt better to the weaning period.

Piglets should not be separated from their mothers for too long periods of time. In the experimental studies conducted by Kuller et al. (2004), in which piglets were separated 12 hours a day for the last eleven days of lactation, up to 22 % of the sows came into heat during this phase. The piglets weighed less at weaning with intermittent suckling, but recovered a good condition more rapidly than the control animals. The sows with which intermittent suckling was used lost less weight at weaning.

At experimental level, some researchers have used intermittent suckling for 12 hours during the first 21 days of lactation to stimulate oestrus in the sows and combine gestation with lactation. However, the results have not been very satisfactory as these oestrus cycles take place so early that they are often anovulatory.

Supplementary feed for piglets

The three-week batch farrowing system does not allow the new cross-fostering systems to be applied correctly in a systematic manner. In some countries such as the Netherlands, piglets are therefore given supplementary feed in addition to the milk provided by the sow. A piglet's growth may be limited by the sow's milk production, so an extra intake of milk increases the growth rate of suckling piglets.

Mixed systems combining the two techniques are increasingly used on very productive farms: cross-fostering and supplementary feeding with formula and other types of supplements.

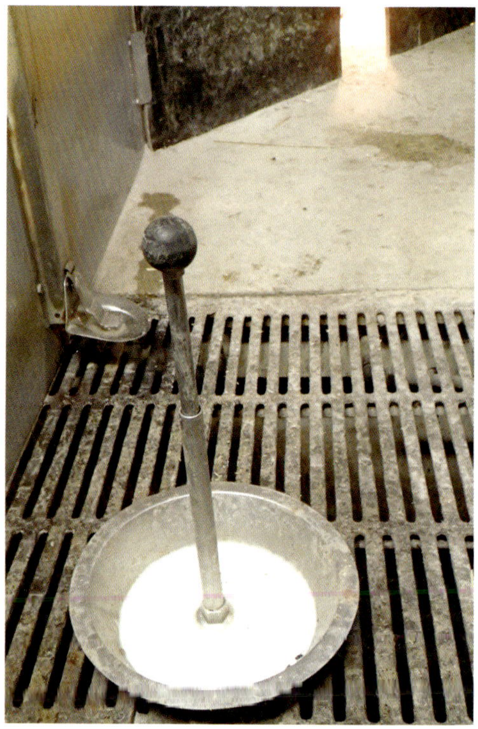

Figure 5 Feeding bowl with milk for small piglets in the farrowing room.

Weaning management

The term **weaning** refers to the time when piglets are separated from their mother and milk is replaced by feed as their main source of nourishment. This time is crucial to ensure piglets have a good start to the transition period and, therefore, to the first phase of the fattening period. It is also an important time for the weaned sow, which will show signs of oestrus 3-5 days later.

Weaning management in piglets

Weaning is a very delicate and stressful time for piglets, as they undergo a series of very important but sudden changes:

- Loss of maternal protection and sudden separation from their mother.
- Transfer to a different rearing site, in many cases accompanied by transportation (sometimes with long journeys).
- Very frequent changes of pen mates, usually with much larger groups than the original litter, with the resulting fights to reestablish hierarchy.
- New feeding systems and feeding and drinking troughs, which piglets must learn to use.
- Cessation of antibody transfer through the sow's milk.
- Transition from a warm, liquid diet to a cold, solid diet.
- Greater water needs. Significant changes in the way they are fed: they change from eating in nursing cycles every 40-60 minutes to having ad libitum access to feed, which, in most cases, they have never tried (sudden contact with vegetable protein).

Separation from the sow is accompanied by typical loud squeals and grunt calls by the piglets, which start immediately after weaning. The frequency and pitch of those calls have been used to measure their stress levels. Piglets weaned at three weeks of age vocalise more than those weaned at four weeks of age.

Weaning management in sows

Sows undergo very significant physiological changes at weaning, and go from milk production to a new oestrus cycle. Cessation of milk production occurs suddenly when the piglets stop nursing and the feed and water should not be rationed in this phase, as it is important for sows to have a good body condition to have good ovulations.

Sows are also moved to a different location on the farm at weaning. They are usually taken to group pens in the service-control area in order to favour the onset of oestrus. In these pens, they are grouped per productive cycle and size so the largest sows let the youngest and smallest ones eat and hierarchy is rapidly reestablished.

Objectives at weaning

Sow

Achieving a good body condition, which will favour:

- A short weaning-to-service interval (WSI).
- A high ovulation rate.

Piglet

Achieving maximum weight at weaning to ensure:

- A lower mortality rate in the first week postweaning.
- A higher average daily gain (ADG) during the transition and fattening periods.

Weaning day

The day of weaning on a farm may vary and depends not only on the logistics of the movement of piglets to the next phase of production (transition, isowean or "wean to finish" systems), but also on how services and farrowings are managed on the farm. For example, a farm that typically weans mainly on Thursdays will have the largest group of services on the Monday and Tuesday of the following week. However, with these services, there will be farrowings on Thursdays and Fridays, which will require more management at weekends.

In the past few years and with the appearance of new hyperprolific genetic lines (with gestations up to 1-2 days longer), some farmers have tended to wean at weekends. The decision to wean on a Saturday or Sunday can lead to services being performed at the end of the week, but farrowings will take place at the beginning of the week, which will allow better care and management of piglets during their first days of life.

Table 1 Correspondence between day of weaning and day of services and farrowings.

Weekly work plan							
Weaning	**Monday**	**Tuesday**	**Wednesday**	**Thursday**	**Friday**	**Saturday**	**Sunday**
Thursday**	Service	Service	Service Farrowing	Farrowing	Farrowing		
Saturday**	Farrowing	Farrowing	Service	Service	Service		Farrowing
Sunday**	Farrowing	Farrowing	Farrowing	Service	Service	Service	

*Recommended for lines with an average of 114 days in gestation.
*Recommended for lines with an average of 115 days in gestation.

Time of weaning

It is better to wean early in the morning. After feeding the sows and without waiting for the piglets to start with the nursing cycles, the piglets should be removed from the sows so the latter can be taken to the service-control area. Oestrus stimulation and contact with the boar should start the next day.

The piglets are then taken to their new location, classified by size and housed in separate pens with an appropriate density. They are taught to eat and drink, shown the water source and given their first meal.

Although it is a standard management practice, it is better not to mix piglets of different litters during the post-weaning period if the facilities allow it (two litters at most can be mixed together). This will favour their growth and reduce the fights that take place when piglets of different mothers are mixed together and have to reestablish their social hierarchy. The post-weaning pens should therefore be small.

Post-weaning housing

It is recommended that the sows are taken to the service and control area at weaning. If this area is in the gestation unit, it should be located in the rows of stalls that have better lighting and allow a better stimulation of oestrus and contact with the boar.

Sows weaned in groups have a shorter weaning-to-oestrus interval than those weaned in stalls, provided appropriate contact with the boar is ensured. However, at a practical level, group housing makes proper sow management and feeding more difficult. This is the reason why, on many operations, sows are weaned in stalls.

The hours of exposure to light are very important in order to avoid seasonal anoestrus. A photoperiod of 14-16 hours at an intensity of 200 lux is recommended. Farms in Northern Europe use rows of fluorescent tubes at a height of one metre above the sows' head (Fig. 6).

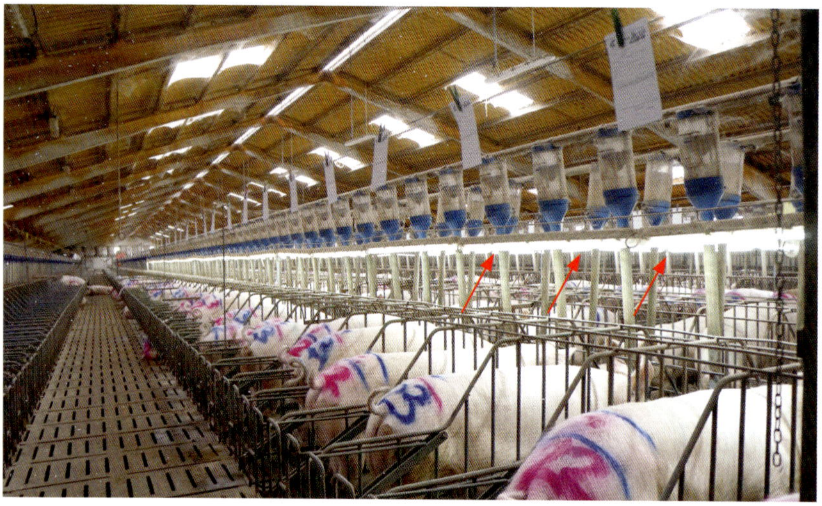

Figure 6 Service and control area with extra lighting (fluorescent tubes, arrows) to favour the onset of oestrus in the sows.

Boar effect

The effect exerted by boars on the reproductive function of sows is well known. Oestrus appears earlier in sows that are in direct contact with the boar after weaning. This contact should start immediately after weaning and last for approximately 20 minutes a day.

The boar should walk in front of the sows and oestrus should not be stimulated in groups of more than 5-6 sows at a time. The use of doors along the aisle of the service and control area is thus recommended, to ensure appropriate contact of the boar with the sows. In addition, it is good to stimulate oestrus with at least two different males, since some sows –either due to rejection or fear– show more signs of oestrus with some boars than with others. Sows with no evident signs of oestrus or that have not come into heat after four or five days should be taken directly to the boar's pen. This should be done for two reasons: it increases sexual stimulation and not all sows show very clear signs of oestrus.

Feeding levels during lactation and at weaning

Feeding is key to ensure sows do not lose body condition and raise piglets with an optimal weight. Feeding levels are influenced by the number of meals (2-3), the composition and digestibility of the diet, the energy it provides, the physical presentation of the feed (sows eat more with liquid feeding), the type of drinking trough and the sows' body condition at farrowing as a result of the feeding practices during gestation. For these reasons, the main objective of feeding in this phase is to achieve the maximum feed intake possible without upsetting the sow.

In order to achieve an appropriate WSI, proper feeding is important both during lactation and at the time of weaning.

There is a direct relationship between feed consumption during lactation and the WSI. The higher the voluntary feed intake, the shorter the WSI. This is more relevant in gilts. An appropriate feed intake during lactation ensures the maintenance of a good body condition. Studies recommend that, during this phase, sows do not lose more than one point with the traditional body condition scoring system, which classifies sows on a scale of 1 to 5 (1 corresponding to very thin sows and 5 to very fat sows), or 3 mm of fat, if an ultrasonic device is used to measure dorsal fat.

In the past few years, **flushing** at weaning has regained relevance. The term flushing refers to the increase in the feeding levels provided to sows in order to stimulate the onset of oestrus and favour a greater ovulation rate. From the day of weaning until the onset of oestrus –when the sows' appetite decreases significantly–, it is recommended that the sows continue to be fed a high-energy feed (flushing feed) or a supplement of approximately 150 g of dextrose. If this option is not possible, the sows should be fed lactation feed. A high feed intake is essential; two daily meals are therefore recommended to achieve intakes of 4-5 kg of feed per sow and day.

There are supplements rich in sugar available on the market, which, in principle, favour an increase in the ovulation rate and ensure much more homogeneous litters at birth due to their beneficial effect on follicle development. These are administered for 3 days before and until 3-4 days after weaning.

> The size of the litter weaned is directly related to the WSI. The larger the number of piglets and the higher their weight, the shorter the WSI.

Variation factors affecting milk production

A sow's lactation curve corresponds to an ascending curve that reaches a peak at approximately week 3 or 4 of lactation and remains high until week 5, to then start a descending phase, with a certain level of persistence, and end with the cessation of milk production at about week 8 or 9.

A sow's milk production depends on her genetic line and, above all, on feeding during lactation. Nevertheless, it is also influenced by:

- Water intake.
- The temperature, humidity levels and ventilation in the farrowing room. Temperatures above 20-24 °C reduce appetite and, consequently, milk production.
- Silence and a quiet environment in the farrowing room.
- Time of the year. Summer, as hot temperatures cause a reduction in milk production.
- Health status of the sow and her piglets.
- Age of the sow. The sows that produce most milk are those that have farrowed three or four times.
- Size of the litter it is nursing.
- Piglet weight at birth and vigour.
- Body condition of the sow. Fat sows at farrowing produce less milk.
- Number and type of functional teats (Fig. 7).

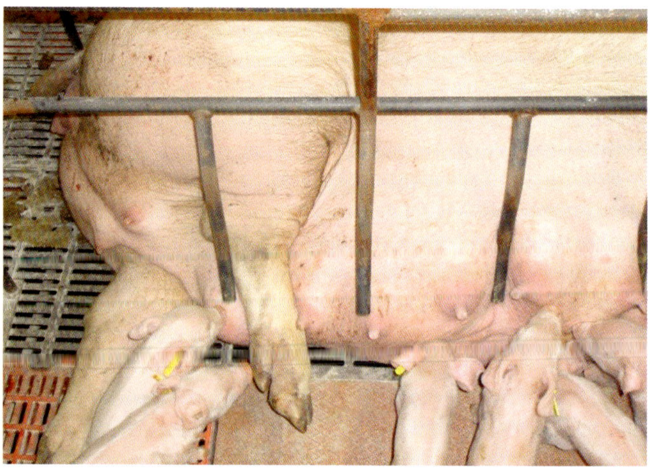

Figure 7 Sow with inguinal mammary glands.

Influence of lactation on productive performance

The weaning-to-service interval (WSI) is greatly influenced by the duration of lactation, particularly by short lactations (Fig. 8). During the lactation period, sows remain in anoestrus since the stimulus of the nursing piglets leads to the secretion of prolactin, which suppresses hormonal activity in the ovary and the start of the oestrus cycle. The duration of the lactation period should provide enough time to ensure proper correct uterine involution, which is the regeneration of the uterus to favour future gestations (Fig. 9). Weaning at less than 18 days of lactation in multiparous sows and at less than 21 days in first-parity sows causes problems in uterine involution, with the resulting increase in the weaning-to-service interval.

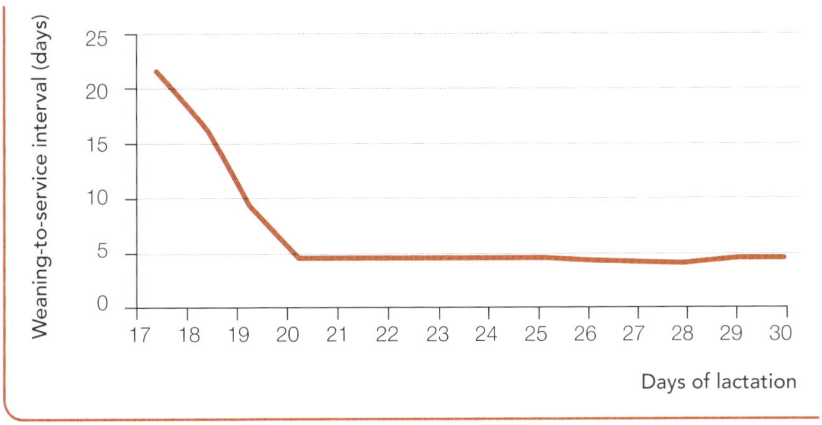

Figure 8 Weaning-to-service interval (WSI) and its relation with the duration of lactation. Adapted from Oliva, J.E. Efficiency in farrowing units. *Fatro seminar*, 2014.

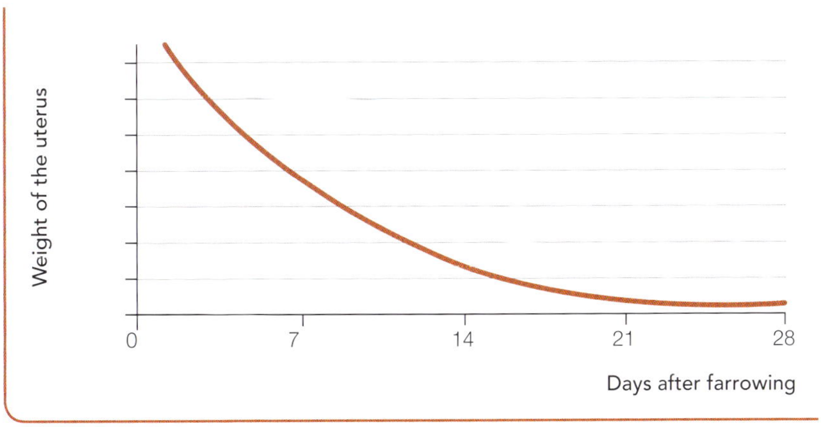

Figure 9 Uterine involution curve after farrowing. Adapted from Whittemore, C.T. *The science and practice of pig production*. Harlow Scientific and Technical Editions, Arlington, 1993.

The WSI may also be longer and anoestrus may even appear when partial weaning or nurse sows are used. This is due to an incorrect uterine involution or, on many occasions, to an onset of oestrus in the farrowing unit during lactation, caused by a reduction in the nursing stimulus by the piglets, which leads to a decrease in prolactin levels and thus triggers the reproductive cycle.

Other factors are affected by the duration of lactation:

- **Onset of oestrus.** The shorter the WSI, the longer the oestrus. Ovulation tends to occur at the end of the oestrus phase. It is important to adjust the insemination protocols based on the WSI.
- **Fertility.** It also declines when age at weaning is reduced. The decrease in fertility is particularly significant when piglets are weaned at less than 20 days of age.
- **Prolificacy.** The size of the litter is usually lower in sows weaned with fewer days of lactation as a result of a lack of uterine involution (which leads to a lower ovulation rate and reduced embryonic survival) (Fig. 10).
- **Piglet weight at weaning.** The longer the lactation period, the heavier the piglets will be at weaning. On average, piglets gain 250 g a day during lactation and about 300 g a day in the last week. In addition, the more piglets are weaned, the lower the average weight at weaning will be. For this reason, some swine genetics companies have, in the past few years, established weaning targets that combine the number of weaned piglets and weight at weaning. Their target is to wean 200 kg of piglet per sow and year.

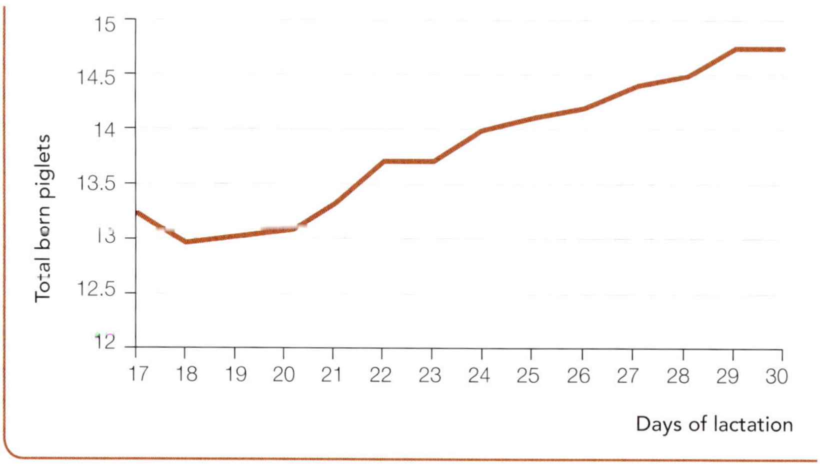

Figure 10 Effect of the duration of lactation on litter size at the next farrowing. Adapted from Oliva, J.E. Efficiency in farrowing units. *Fatro seminar*, 2014.

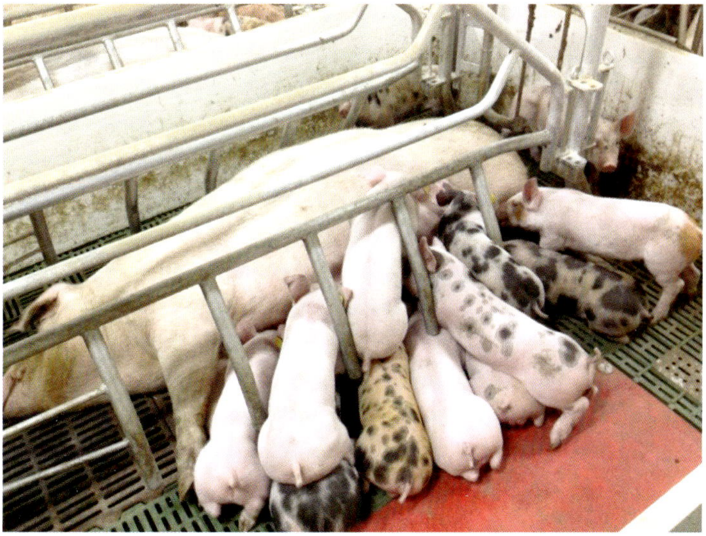

Figure 11 Piglets that will be weaned at 28 days of age and more than 9 kg of live weight. *Image courtesy of Salvador Batalle.*

- **Productive life of the sow.** Sows with short lactations will produce more litters per year than sows with long lactations. However, they will give rise a higher percentage of sows culled earlier than expected due to a higher metabolic demand.

Advantages and disadvantages of early weaning

Advantages	Disadvantages
Larger number of farrowings/sow/year due to shorter lactation periods.	The lower the piglet's weight, the more its viability is compromised.
Greater rotation in the farrowing units due to shorter lactation periods. The number of farrowing places required is therefore lower, which reduces costs, as these places are the most expensive on a swine operation.	Environmental requirements are stricter in piglets weaned early. Special facilities, feeding and management practices are necessary.
From a health point of view, piglets are weaned with a better health status, since some diseases of sows are not transmitted to piglets at very early ages.	When small piglets are weaned, they need to spend more time in the transition area, which will therefore need to be larger.
	From the point of view of the sow, early weaning means little time is allowed for uterine involution to take place correctly.

Types of weaning depending on piglet age

According to the current European legislation on animal welfare, piglets should not be weaned under 28 days of age, unless a veterinary practitioner recommends they are weaned earlier as an extraordinary measure for the control and/or eradication of a disease, and provided they are taken to facilities specially prepared for this purpose.

In the past few years and for health and management reasons, the tendency was to wean at less than 21 days of age, especially as a result of the works of Tom Alexander and Hank Harris, from the universities of Cambridge and Iowa respectively. Both developed a theory, or **isowean principle** (isolated weaning), which aims at controlling the transmission of many diseases from sows to their piglets.

The isowean principle involves producing piglets free from specific pathogenic agents. This is achieved through **early**, **medicated** (with medicated feed to eradicate specific bacterial diseases) and **segregated** (piglets are separated from their mother when they still have high maternal antibody levels) weaning. These theories revolutionised swine production worldwide and some of the ideas and concepts they introduced are still relevant. For instance, they favoured early weaning at less than 21 days of age in order to prevent the transmission of many diseases from sows to their piglets (Table 3).

These theories have evolved and, both for animal welfare reasons and to achieve a heavier weaning weight and better uterine involution, the tendency is now moving towards weaning at 28 days of age, with better prolificacy and fertility results. Nonetheless, many operations still wean on average at 24-25 days of age.

Taking into account the high levels of stress experienced by piglets at weaning, the older and heavier they are, the better they will overcome them. In addition, their enzymatic and digestive systems will be more developed, which is important for the transition to a feed-based diet.

Ultra-early weaning (5-8 days of age)

This method is only applied in programmes of pathogen eradication in combination with "all-in, all-out" strategies, in segregated weaning and with antibiotic therapies. Piglets are usually fed a liquid and warm diet in special rooms for the first few days. The diets administered are usually rich in milk.

Table 3 Segregated early weaning. Maximum age at weaning in a segregated location to prevent the transmission of endemic pathogens to piglets. Muirhead, M.R. and Alexander, T.J.L. *Managing Pig Health and the Treatment of Disease*. 5M Enterprises, Sheffield, UK, 1997.

Infection/disease	Age (days)	Medication/vaccination for greater safety
Actinobacillus pleuropneumoniae (APP)	< 28	Medication
Aujeszky's disease virus	21	Vaccination
Bordetella bronchiseptica	5	Medication+Vaccination
Swine influenza virus	16	None
Mycoplasma hyopneumoniae (EP)	10	Medication+Vaccination
Pasteurella multocida (toxigenic) (AR)	8-10	Medication+Vaccination
PRCV	<14 (NK)	None
PRRS virus	<16 (NR)	None
Coccidia	–	Not possible
E. coli	–	Not possible
Internal parasites	< 14	Medication
Parvovirus	< 28	Vaccination
Swine dysentery	< 21	Medication
TGE	21 (NK)	None

APP: *Actinobacillus pleuropneumoniae*; EP: enzootic pneumonia; AR: atrophic rhinitis; PRCV: porcine respiratory coronavirus; TGE: transmissible gastroenteritis; PED: porcine epidemic diarrhoea; NR: non-reliable; NK: not known

The main disadvantage of ultra-early weaning is that it does not allow enough time for the sow's uterus to involute completely.

Partial weaning of the strongest piglets may be performed once these have ingested colostrum, between days 1 and 3 (see Chapter Nutrition), but this should only be done with surplus piglets and the sow should not be weaned.

Standard weaning at 3 weeks of age

This has been the standard age at weaning in the past years and piglets are still weaned at that age on many operations with two- or three-week batch farrowing.

With an average age at weaning of 21 days (and an interval ranging from 18 to 23 days), many sows are weaned at 18 days. This is detrimental to uterine involution and causes a decrease in productive performance in the following reproductive cycle.

Weaning at 28 days of age

It is the most recommended age at weaning for several reasons. Most of them have already been explained, but the main reason is that a higher weaning weight is achieved. As a result, piglets are able to eat earlier in the post-weaning period, have a faster growth rate and fewer digestive problems at weaning, as their enzymatic and intestinal activity are more developed. All this significantly reduces mortality.

Weaning at 4 weeks of age increases the feed intake of piglets in the lactation period, which results in lower stress levels at weaning.

There is a clear positive relationship between weight at weaning and weight at slaughter (Table 4).

When weaning takes place at 28 days of age on average, some sows are weaned at 21 days and have a second lactation to nurse a second litter for 14 more days. The sows that can be weaned after 21 days are those whose piglets have an appropriate weight and those that are losing body condition.

It is cheaper to produce kilograms of piglets when these are fed by their mother to achieve a higher weaning weight than when they are given feed and other nutritional supplements.

Table 4 Influence of weight at birth on weaning weight and growth during the fattening period until slaughter. Adapted from Pluske, J.R. et al. *Weaning the pig. Concepts and consequences* Wageningen Academic Publishers. The Netherlands, 2003.

Influence of weight at birth (higher weight against lower weight) and weaning weight on feed intake and growth until slaughter			
		Higher weight	Lower weight
Weight (kg)	• Birth	1.83	1.30
	• Weaning (20 d)	6.6	5.7
Weaning up to 110 kg	• ADG (g/d)	1,866	1,783
	• ADG (g/d)	851	796

ADI: average daily intake; ADG: average daily gain.

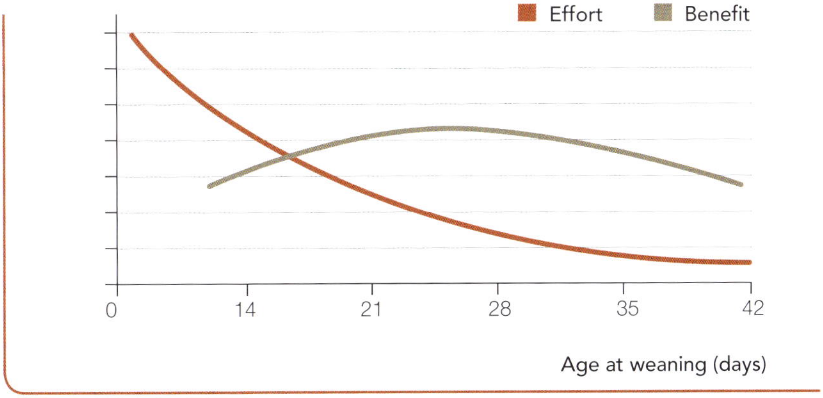

Figure 12 Curve of effort and benefit, showing how it is best to wean piglets at 28 days of age. Adapted from Whittemore, C.T. *The science and practice of pig production*. Harlow Scientific and Technical Editions, Arlington, 1993.

Partial weaning

Partial weaning involves removing a small number of piglets from a litter so the sow ends the lactation period with a better body condition. This is usually done between the third and fourth week of lactation, depending on the weaning age and strategy of each farm. With this technique, two or three of the heaviest piglets are weaned in litters of more than 12-14 piglets (10-11 piglets are left), two or four days before weaning. This allows the other piglets in the litter to grow at a faster pace, as they do not have to compete with the strongest piglets (already weaned) and also helps the sow not to lose too much body condition due to a very high demand of milk from the largest piglets and the resulting increase in milk production.

This practice should only be used seven days before weaning and on operations where piglets are weaned at 28 days of age, in order to obtain piglets with a minimum weight that will make them viable in the post-weaning period. Partial weaning is less effective when applied in short lactations of about 21 days. A maximum of two or three piglets per litter should be weaned and the sows should not be left with less than ten piglets. If the piglets' suckling effect (main stimulating factor for the production of prolactin and for a good milk production) is suddenly reduced, there is a risk –which is greater for some genetic lines– that the sow may come in heat while in lactation. Farmers often do not detect this onset of oestrus during lactation and some sows do not come in heat as expected after weaning, which causes problems at the time of service and long weaning-to-service intervals. On other occasions, the cause is an extremely early onset of oestrus, in the first three days post-weaning.

Some studies show that partial weaning in first and second-parity gilts in long lactations leads to a reduction in the WSI, a greater prolificacy in the next farrowing and to better fertility.

Partial weaning in short lactations can lead to extremely early onsets of oestrus and heat detection problems, as well as to an increase in the WSI.

Oestrus in lactation

If the suckling effect is considerably reduced for any reasons, oestrus sometimes appears during the lactation period while the sow is still producing milk. It is more common than it seems, especially on operations with genetic lines prone to this type of oestrus. In these cases, the sows' behaviour and feed intake should be monitored at the end of lactation, since sows in oestrus in this phase do not eat in the same way as weaned sows do.

The environment of the farrowing unit does not allow sows to show clear signs of oestrus, especially if the farm personnel does not expect them.

Some of the causes that may lead to oestrus in lactation are given next:

- Death of a high percentage of piglets in the litter from the seventh day postpartum.
- Overfeeding, particularly with several meals a day.
- Partial weaning of more than 2-3 piglets, usually among the largest ones, which are removed seven days before weaning. A decline in the amount of milk demanded may result in oestrus 3-5 days later.
- Placing several litters together before the weaning period, which results in the sow not being sufficiently "milked" in group suckling.
- Prolonged lactations, in particular if the sow is used as a nurse sow of a much younger litter (less demanding and with a lower suckling capacity).
- Problems of agalactia.
- Piglets provided with supplementary feed, so that their demand for milk is considerably reduced.
- Prolonged intermittent lactations.
- Any other process leading to a drop in the demand for milk.

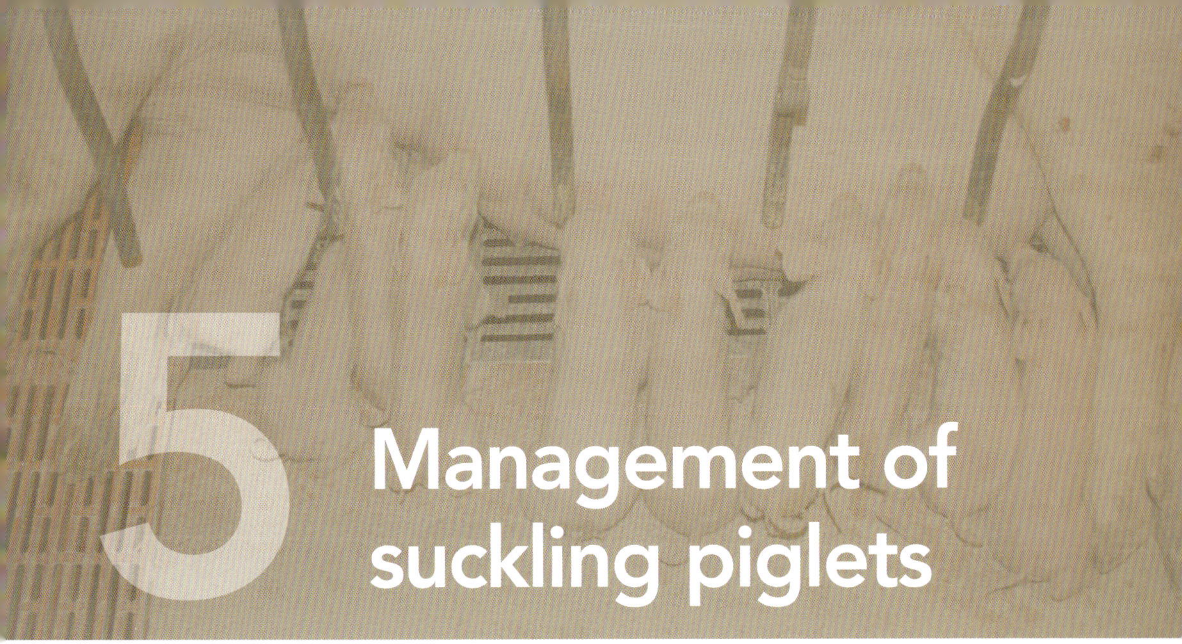

5 Management of suckling piglets

The goal of piglet management in the farrowing unit is to achieve a high weaning weight and high health status for the largest possible number of animals. An appropriate environment and optimal management practices are essential to reach this goal and ensure piglets are prepared to cope with weaning without suffering from severe stress problems.

Piglets weaned at about 21 days of age should weigh more than 6-6.5 kg, while those weaned at 28 days should weigh between 8 and 9 kg.

This chapter addresses the key aspects to maximise newborn piglet survival, as well as other important factors to obtain piglets with a correct weight and health status at the time of weaning. It also includes a review of the importance of colostrum and of the main treatments administered to piglets during their processing to prevent certain diseases.

Birth-to-weaning mortality

Birth-to-weaning deaths contribute to most of the pig losses occurring between thc time when they are born and that when they are sold. More than half of the total deaths on an operation occur in the piglets' first days of life. The objective of producing the largest number of kilograms of meat per sow and year is therefore greatly affected by these deaths and the operation's total production costs are increased while its profitability is reduced.

Management practices aimed at providing optimal care to piglets in their first hours of life are undoubtedly the best way of reducing pre-weaning mortality.

Approximately 12-13 % of piglets die in the period from birth to weaning (in 2013, the figures from BDporc –a data bank on Spanish pig production– indicate an average of 12.14 %). This percentage can now be reduced to 4-5 % on the best farms, where farrowing unit management is excellent, especially with regard to farrowings. However, these percentages have increased due to the appearance of new hyperprolific lines with very large litters, which are more heterogeneous in size and weight and may include a higher number of non-viable piglets at birth. Proper nurse sow and cross-fostering management is key to solve this situation.

Starvation, hypothermia, crushing, diarrhoea and low viability at birth are among the main causes of mortality in this period. These causes can represent more than 80 % of the deaths of newborn piglets. These generally occur in the first three days of life.

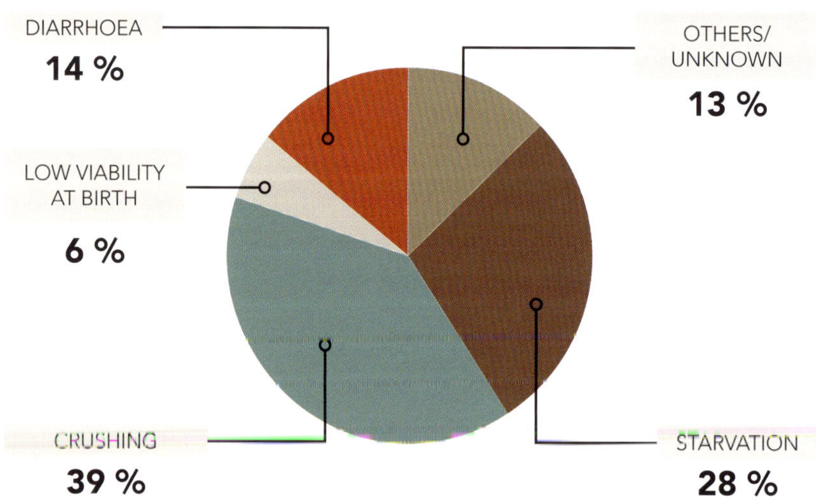

Figure 1 Causes of death in the period from birth to weaning.

The factors contributing to piglet vitality and survival can be classified into:

- Factors inherent to the parents (breeding sow and boar).
- Factors inherent to the piglet.
- Factors associated with the personnel who monitor farrowings and are in charge of taking care of the piglets.
- Factors depending the breeding sow's diet.
- Factors related to environmental control practices and farm facilities.

In order to prevent early postpartum deaths, it is necessary to ensure piglets get a sufficient amount of colostrum and to provide them with areas of thermal comfort to prevent heat and energy losses. Good management practices should also be followed to reduce early exposure to pathogens, as well as correct fostering protocols to increase their chances of survival.

Farrowings should be monitored. If they are induced, qualified personnel should be present to monitor the process.

A good colostrum intake is vital during the farrowing process and in the following hours.

Most sows remain in recumbent position; the top row of teats is therefore often the only one to be exposed. Multiparous sows may also have very large mammary glands, which makes access to their teats more difficult to small piglets. A limited number of exposed teats is a hindrance to appropriate colostrum intake by all the piglets in a litter.

Moreover, piglets are born with no humoral protection and their body only contains enough fat and energy reserves for a single day of life. They cannot regulate their inner body temperature until a few days after birth, so that anything causing a reduction in colostrum and milk production or consumption will compromise their health and growth.

Humid environments, cold floors or low environmental temperatures lead to piglets consuming glucose more rapidly and using up their glycogen reserves. An inadequate milk intake will thus cause their death. In addition, piglets have a large body surface in relation to their weight and lose more heat than adult pigs.

The causes of pre-weaning mortality, especially in the first days after birth, are summarised in Figure 2.

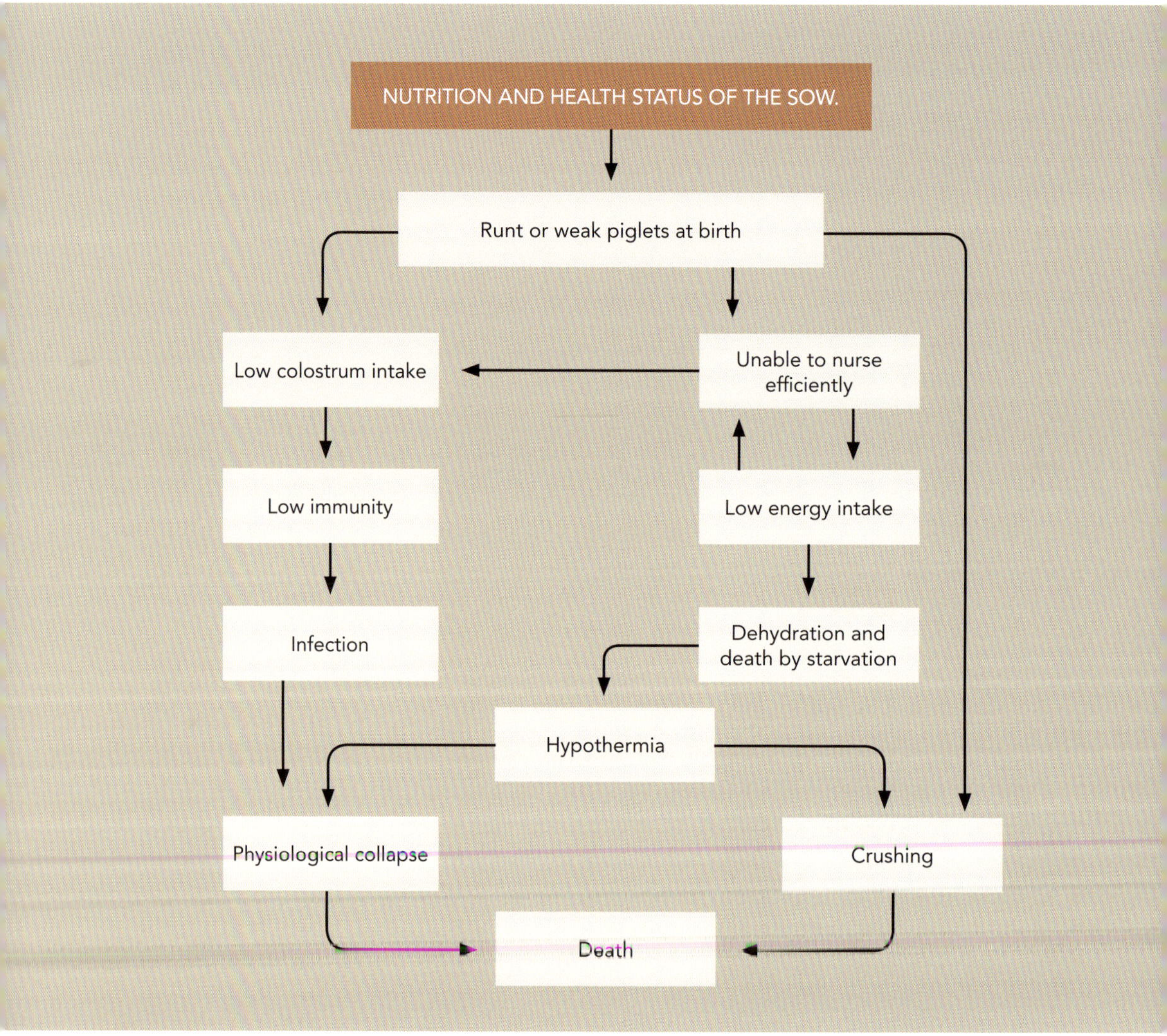

Figure 2 Relationships between the different causes of mortality before weaning. From Mackinnon, J.D. Manejo predestete de los lechones: estrategias para la supervivencia, salud y crecimiento (II). *Avances.* Volume VI, April 2009.

Another key point is weight at birth, since a piglet's chances of survival are greater if its weight at birth is within the appropriate range. In addition to several crucial factors during the gestation period (correct feeding of the sows, etc.), genetics companies use weight at birth as an element to take into account, as it is, together with survival, an inheritable factor. Weight at birth is extremely important nowadays, as genetic improvements and new hyperprolific lines have given rise to sows with a larger number of piglets per farrowing, but heterogeneity and weight variability within litters have considerably increased.

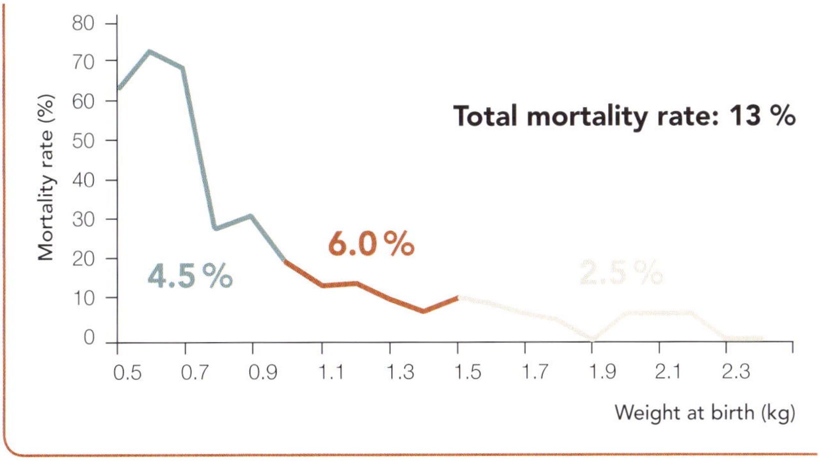

Figure 3 Relation between weight at birth and mortality rate. From Thorup, F. www.porkcrc.com.au/Flemming_Thorup.ppt.

Weight gain is essential to maintain body temperature above thermoneutrality (35-36 °C) and build body fat reserves. A piglet's chances of survival are thus considerably higher if it is able to increase its live weight by 10 % on its first day of life.

> It has been demonstrated that up to 70 % of piglets with a weight below 600 g die in the first 24 hours after birth.

To control these factors, it is necessary to ensure that:

- Genetic programmes optimise newborn piglet survival and maximise weight at birth.
- Nipple drinkers work correctly and have a sufficient water flow for sows and piglets.
- Feed troughs and dispensers are in good condition.
- Anti-crushing systems are in good condition and properly adjusted.
- Piglets are mature at birth.
- Farrowing pens are comfortable and clean.
- Ventilation and heating systems are inspected regularly and fully functional.
- Animals are appropriately distributed in the unit.
- Sow body condition is adequate.
- Sows are healthy and any individual showing signs of disease or possible infection is treated rapidly.
- The sows' udders are in good condition. Their teats are functional.
- The sows' records and clinical histories are up-to-date and the data collected are reliable. It is necessary to know how many piglets each sow can nurse based on previous records.
- The personnel should be trained and motivated. Work protocols should be clear and precise (cross-fostering techniques, alternate nursing, etc.).

Another concept that should be borne in mind, in particular with hyperprolific lines, is the number of live piglets on day 5 postpartum, due to the high birth-to-weaning mortality rate originally shown by these lines. Selection of maternal lines has changed over time and, although it used to be based almost only on prolificacy, other characteristics have started to be taken into account in the past few years, such as life span, conformation, viability of the litter and number of live piglets on day 5 postpartum. These aspects have been considered key to achieve, by means of genetic selection, highly productive animals that are adapted to the reality of swine operations.

Colostrum and importance of an appropriate intake

Sows secrete colostrum immediately after birth. Colostrum is rich in proteins and immunoglobulins and is a source of highly digestible nutrients, which are very important for newborn piglets to survive. It also contains growth factors that are essential to organ development.

A sow's milk has lower protein and immunoglobulin G levels than her colostrum. Nevertheless, it has higher levels of fat, lactose and immunoglobulins A.

> Remarkably, the sow's parity and the size of the litter do not seem to affect milk composition.

The main function of colostrum is to provide piglets with energy and passive immunity, but it also plays an important role in the development of the gastrointestinal tract of newborn piglets.

Colostrum intake is directly correlated with piglet survival in the first hours of life (Fig. 4).

Protein levels in colostrum are high, mainly because of the presence of immunoglobulins. IgG predominate during the first six hours and decrease as lactation progresses. It is important to remember that if farrowing is induced too early, IgG levels will be lower than those expected when gestation has reached full term (Fig. 5).

Piglets obtain amino acids from casein, which is also in charge of transporting calcium and participates in mineral absorption. Another source of aminoacids for piglets is serum proteins. These include albumins and immunoglobulins –which are responsible for passive immunity and the transport of vitamins– and some physiological regulators such as hormone and growth factors.

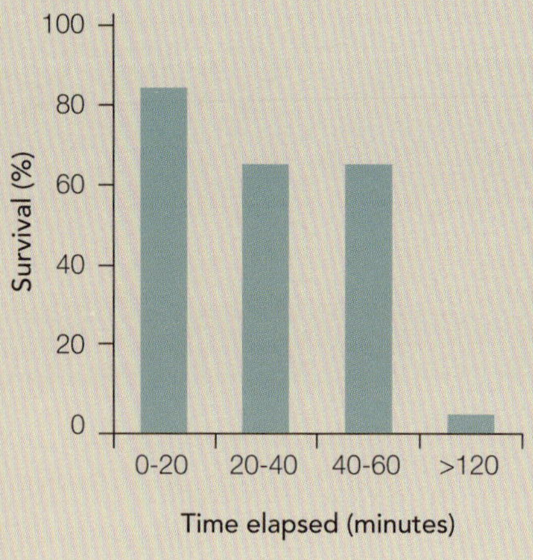

Figure 4 Minutes elapsed between birth and first colostrum feeding and relationship with survival rate. From Palomino, A. *Av. Technol. porc.* 4, 2007.

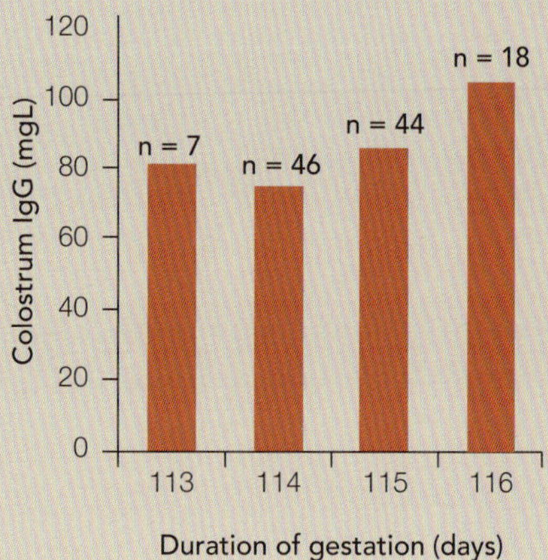

Figure 5 Colostrum IgG levels according to the duration of gestation.From Gin et al., 2008, unpublished data. Cited by Martineau, J.P. and Badouard, B. *London Swine Conference*, 2009.

Fat levels in colostrum are lower than those in milk. They increase from 5 % on day 1 to 13 % on day 3 of lactation, and then go down to 6 % at the end of this period. Colostrum also has a higher concentration in vitamins.

Piglets are born without any immunoglobulins circulating in their blood, as the placenta is epithelio-chorial in pigs and does not allow the transfer of immunity to the foetus in utero. The newborn piglet's bloodstream receives maternal humoral immunity thanks to the ingestion of colostrum in the first hours following its birth. Ingesting colostrum with appropriate amounts of IgG, IgA and IgM is essential, as these immunoglobulins protect piglets from enteric and systemic diseases once they are absorbed through the intestinal barrier.

Immunoglobulin levels in colostrum rapidly decrease after birth and are down by up to 30 % 12 hours after the first piglet is born. It is therefore essential to ensure piglets receive an appropriate amount of colostrum in their first hours of life.

> The efficacy of colostrum to protect a newborn piglet depends on the amount that has been ingested, on its immunoglobulin concentration and on the piglet's intestinal absorptive capacity.

Immunoglobulin absorption through the piglet's intestinal wall is high until 8-12 hours postpartum, but intestinal permeability progressively decreases and is almost non-existent 24 hours after birth.

Colostrum production is highly variable. An average production of 3.5 kg in the first 24 hours of life can be considered, but the range is very wide (from 2 to 6 kg). It should be highlighted that colostrum production does not increase with the weight and size of the litter, so the amount of colostrum available is lower as the number of live-born piglets increases. Accordingly, in hyperprolific sows or in the case of very large litters, it is essential to monitor farrowings and use alternate nursing techniques.

The purpose of sow management should be to enable them to produce an appropriate amount of colostrum/milk for their piglets to guarantee their survival and rapid growth. A sow's milk production peaks in the third week postpartum approximately and decreases from that moment on. The reduced milk production is made up for with feed to obtain heavier piglets at weaning.

Alternate nursing

Alternate nursing is a technique aimed at reducing preweaning mortality; it is used to control colostrum intake and ensure it is sufficient, especially in the case of very large litters. The intervention of the farm personnel reduces the time elapsed between birth and colostrum consumption, minimises the drop in body temperature and increases the probability of all the piglets getting enough colostrum.

It is not a difficult technique, although it requires dedication from the farm personnel. However, the effort is undoubtedly worthwhile. To do so, once a sow has started to farrow, her piglets are monitored and those that have already consumed colostrum are placed away in a warm area, so that those that have not nursed yet can do it without having to compete with the others. The piglets that have been placed in the warm area away from the others may be reintroduced in the group or swapped with those that are nursing after one or two hours. This way, colostrum distribution is more equitable and effective and, what is even more important, the smallest or weakest piglets have greater options to ingest colostrum and therefore to survive. (Figs. 6, 7 and 8).

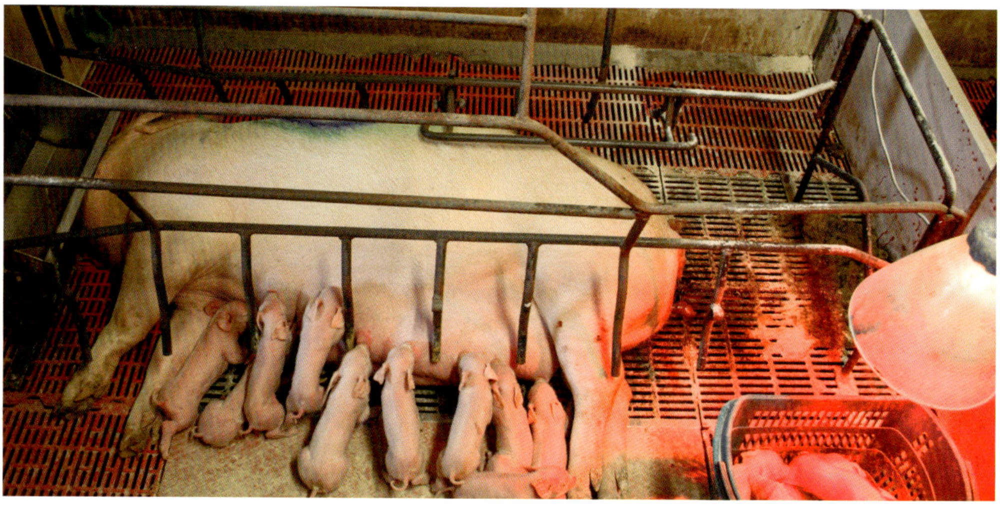

Figure 6 Alternate nursing technique.

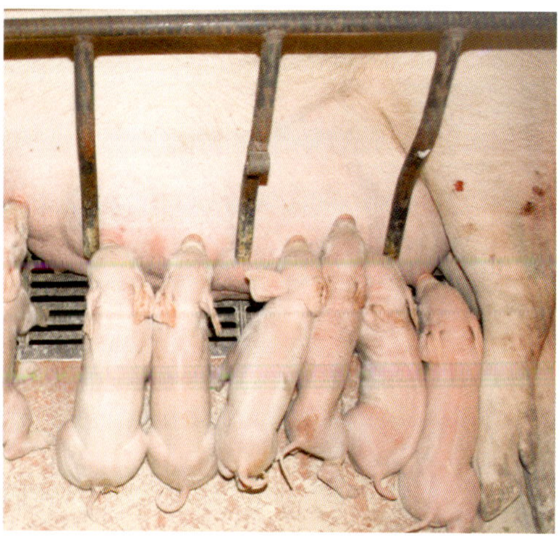

Figure 7 Piglets nursing with no competition.

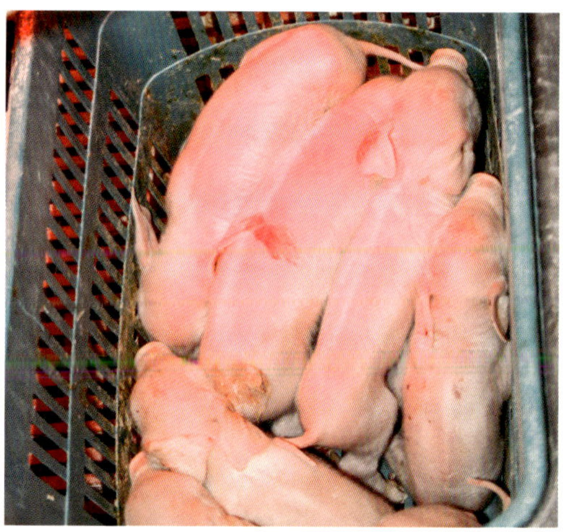

Figure 8 Piglets waiting to nurse.

> **Alternate nursing involves boxing part of the piglets away close to a heat source in turns to ensure appropriate colostrum intake by all the piglets.**

There are two ways of doing it:

- If farrowing is complete, box the largest piglets away so the smallest ones can drink colostrum, and help them to do so if necessary.
- If farrowing is monitored, newborn piglets are placed in a warm area so they do not suffer from hypothermia and those piglets that were born earlier and have already recovered their body temperature are placed with the sow to nurse.

The piglets should be kept away for approximately one hour and a half and those that have had enough colostrum should be marked with a marker or spray.

Routine and specific treatments of piglets

There are two important legal aspects related to the European law on animal welfare to bear in mind in the farrowing house:

- Piglets cannot be weaned before 28 days of life. Weaning at 21 days is only allowed if piglets are taken to facilities that are specially prepared for this purpose.
- With regard to mutilations, tail docking and teeth clipping are not allowed to be performed on a routine basis, but only if there is evidence that, despite having taken all the necessary measures, it has not been possible to prevent injuries to the ears or tails of other pigs or to the teats of the sows. If piglets are castrated after seven days of life, only a veterinary surgeon will be allowed to perform the procedure, using anaesthesia and analgesia.

The husbandry procedures and routine treatments to which piglets are subjected include teeth clipping, disinfection and tying-off of the umbilical cord, identification of the animals and administration of coccidiostatic drugs. On occasions, these procedures also include the treatment of piglets with splay leg, castration, the administration of supplementary nutrients and other treatments, individual weighing of the piglets or whole litter, etc. The order of application of these treatments will vary according to the preferences of the farm workers or will depend on technical or veterinary criteria.

Some operations do not apply all these procedures or postpone them until piglets are three or four days old, so they do not get too stressed. However, processing one-day old piglets is more convenient as they weigh less and are easier to handle. Nonetheless, on farms where mortality rates during the lactation period are high (more than 15 %), it is best to postpone tail docking, teeth clipping and castration for a few days (at least in the smallest individuals).

The best, whenever possible, is to postpone piglet processing until their third day of life, or, at least, until 24 hours after the last batch of sows has farrowed. This way, the atmosphere in the unit is quieter and allows sows to farrow more easily. Piglets are thus more viable, cope better with stress and their colostrum intake is not affected.

Ideally, piglet processing should be postponed until the third day of life, or at least until 24 hours after the last batch of sows has farrowed.

Ideally, piglets should be held so that tail docking, teeth clipping, disinfection of the umbilical cord and iron administration can be performed rapidly, with no need to repeatedly change their position (Fig. 9).

Trolleys can be used to process piglets. These must be clean and disinfected prior to processing each batch. Multi-treatment trolleys that automate some of these tasks are now available on the market. They are very useful on operations with a large number of sows (Figs. 10 and 11). All the material necessary to process piglets should be clean and in perfect condition, in order to minimise the risk of infections, especially with *E.coli.*

After using needles in a litter, these should be placed in a container with a disinfectant, dried and prepared to be used again, provided they are still in good condition and sharp.

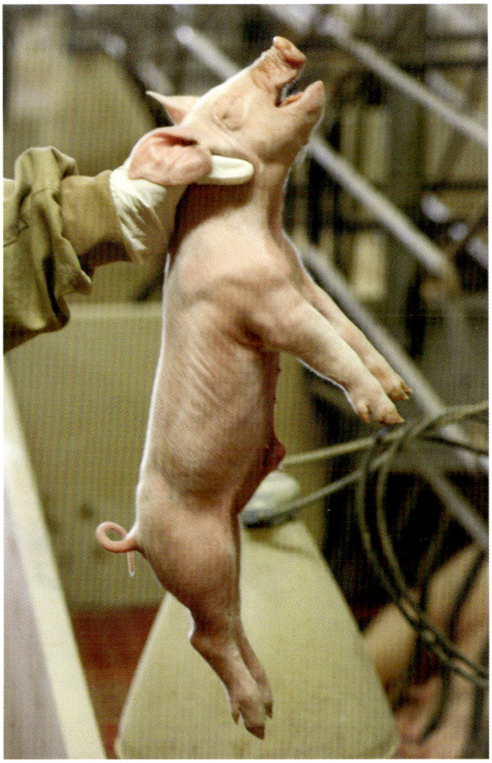

Figure 9 Correct way of holding a piglet for its processing.

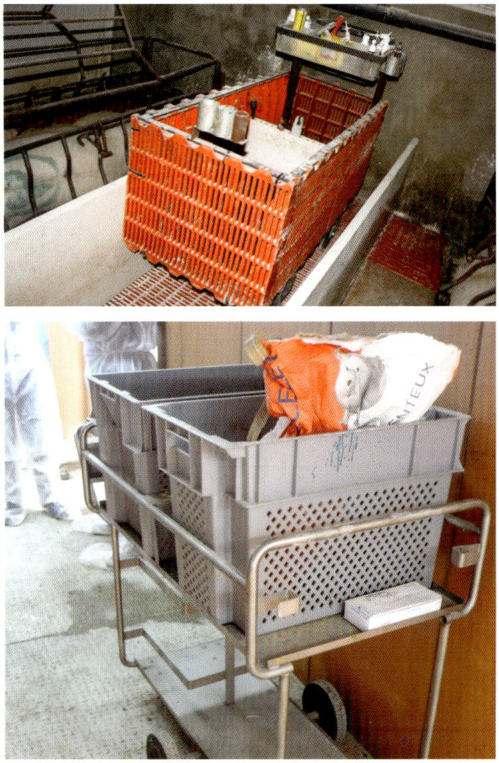

Figure 10 Trolley to process piglets.

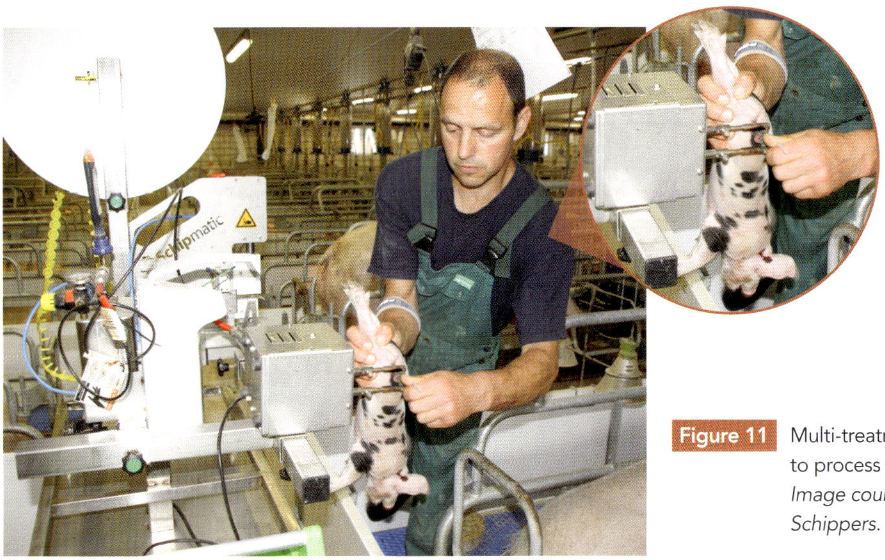

Figure 11 Multi-treatment trolley to process piglets. *Image courtesy of Schippers.*

Piglet processing and routine treatments

Tail docking

Tail docking is performed to ensure pigs are not tail bitten when housed in groups. It should only be done when the different causes of the bites have been investigated (generally in the last phase of the transition and fattening periods) and different protocols have been implemented to prevent them with no positive results.

The procedure is performed in the first few days of life as it is less stressful for piglets, the environment is more hygienic (the farrowing pen is clean when farrowing starts) and piglets have high passive immunity levels thanks to colostrum.

Only instruments especially intended for this purpose should be used. In addition to being cut, the tail should be cauterised to prevent subsequent bleeding and contamination with pathogens (Fig. 12).

The tail should be left at approximately one third of its length (Figs. 13 and 14). If it is cut in excess, it may be too close to the anus and cause an increase in rectal prolapses or infections leading to paralysis of the hindquarters. On the other hand, if it is left too long, bites will not be prevented.

On selective breeding or multiplication farms, the tail is left longer in female piglets (future breeders) to facilitate their handling when they are adults, as their tails allow farm workers to handle them more easily.

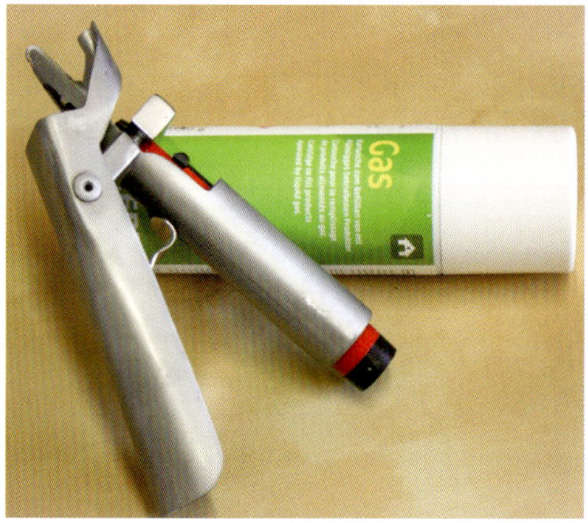

Figure 12 Instruments necessary for tail docking.

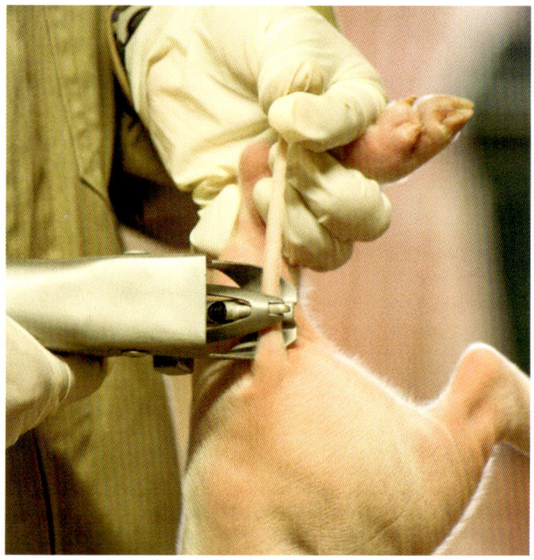

Figure 13 Tail docking.

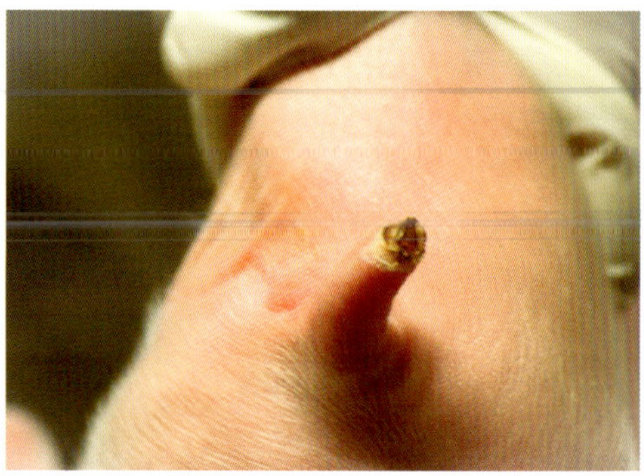

Figure 14 Docked tail.

A few days after having docked the piglet's tail, it is perfectly cauterised and there are no remaining signs of the injury caused by the process.

If teeth clippers are used, the blades should be perfectly sharpened and cleaned between litters.

The same instrument should never be used to clip teeth and dock tails –a common practice on some operations– in order to prevent pathogen transmission, especially digestive pathogens, between the two areas.

Piglet identification

The purpose is to identify piglets permanently in order to record individual parameters in genetic selection programmes or to allow traceability as part of routine production programmes.

The most commonly used techniques are ear tagging and tattooing. However, some countries (e.g. Denmark) use an ear-notching system according to a predefined code that assigns a number to all future breeders from birth.

- Ear tagging is performed using different types of tags available on the market, which will remain with the pig for life.
- Tattoing is carried out with pliers that contain the code to be assigned to the animal. The code is formed by sharpened individual pieces, which, after being dipped in ink, are pressed against the animal's skin to create the tattoo.

Teeth clipping

Newborn piglets have eight very sharp teeth located in the upper and lower mandibles. They sometimes have to be shortened to prevent injuries to the sow's teats during the lactation period or to their litter mates. They should not be cut close to the gums to avoid injuries that may lead to bacterial infections. Care must also be taken not to cause injuries to the tongue.

The current tendency is not to clip teeth or to only do so when detecting that sows do not nurse their piglets well as a consequence of painful teats or worsening of exudative epidermitis, or due to facial necrobacillosis in piglets.

EAR TAGGING

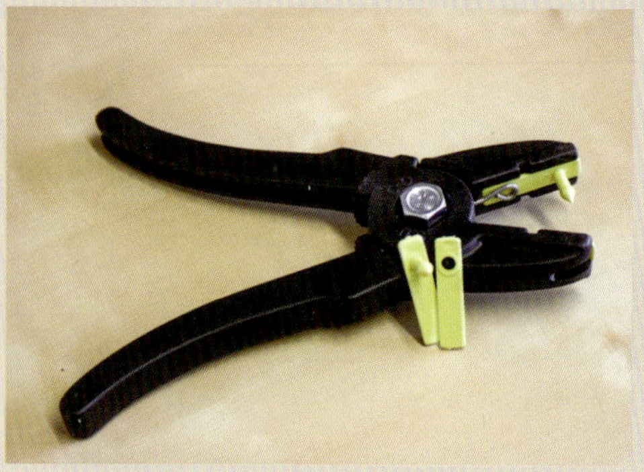

Figure 15 Materials necessary: ear tagger and tags.

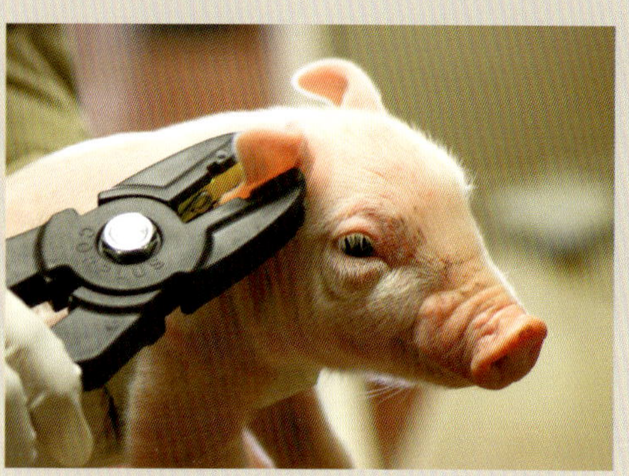

Figure 16 Piglet ear-tagging process.

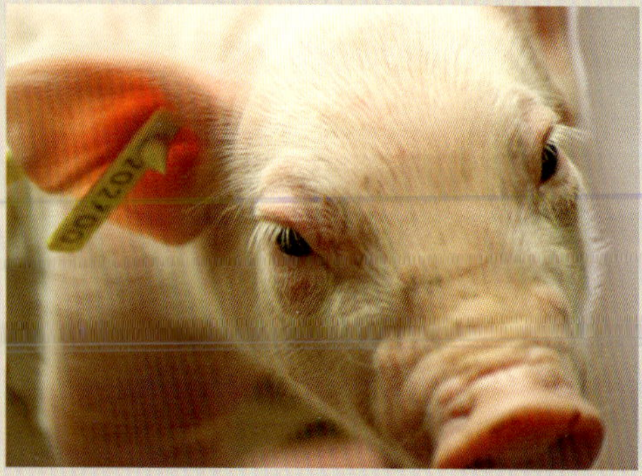

Figure 17 Piglet with an ear tag.

TATTOOING

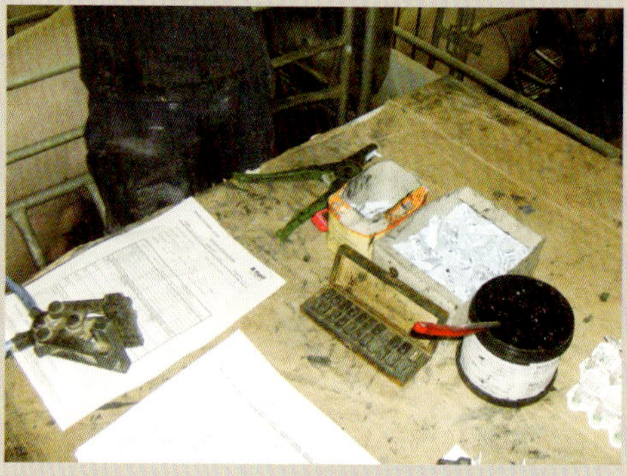

Figure 18 Equipment for tattooing. *Image courtesy of Luis Laborda (Hypor).*

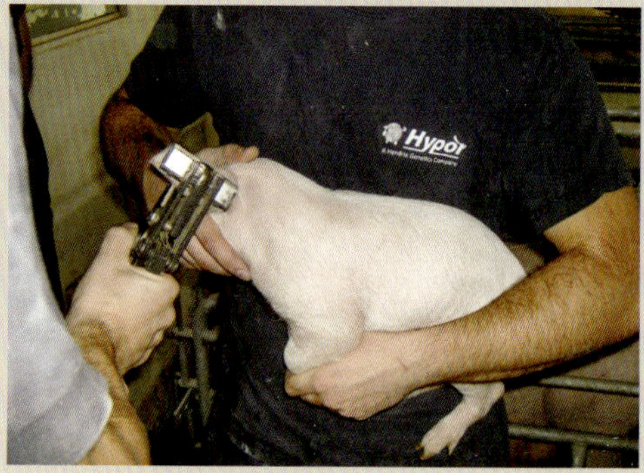

Figure 19 Procedure. *Image courtesy of Luis Laborda (Hypor).*

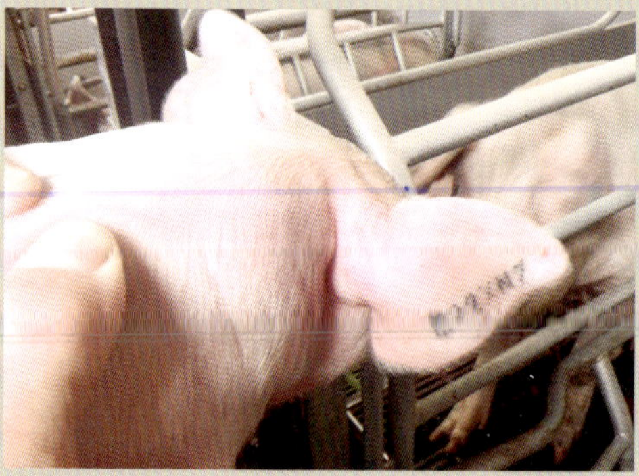

Figure 20 Tattooed piglet.

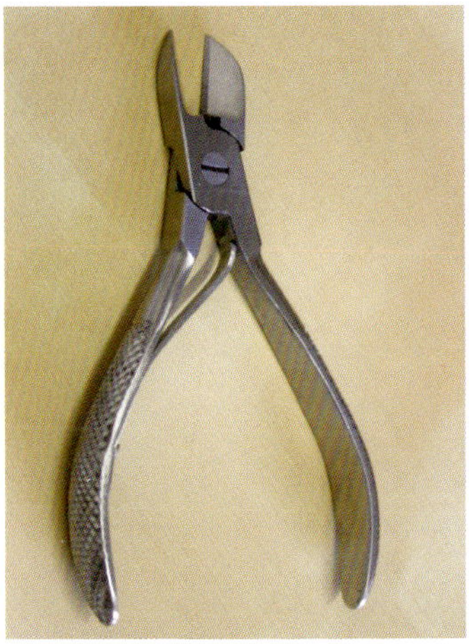

Figure 21 Teeth clippers.

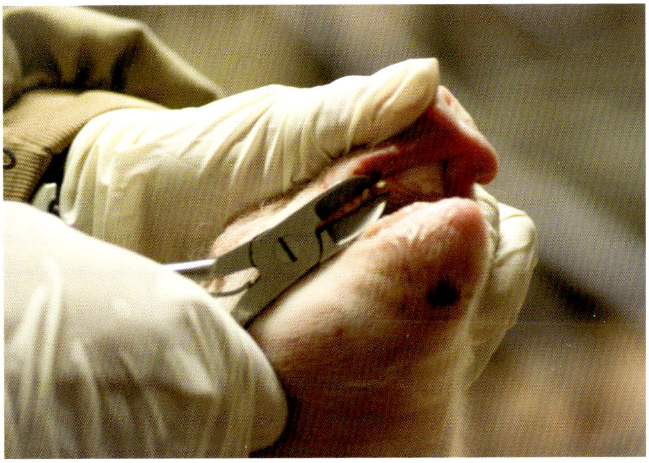

Figure 22 Teeth clipping.

Very sharp teeth clippers are needed to perform this procedure. The blades should be in perfect condition, with no signs of wear. Cutting the whole tooth is not necessary; reducing it to half its length is enough. This will prevent injuries to the piglet's mouth that may hinder nursing. Clipping should be done perpendicular to the orientation of the tooth and in a clean manner, so the tooth is not chipped.

Since the mouth is a source of bacteria, clippers should be disinfected between litters. Teeth grinders are effective, but their use is complicated and the time dedicated to this process is considerably increased.

Iron administration

Piglet frequently suffer from iron deficiency anaemia. Iron is the primary component of the haem group, which in turn is one of the elements of haemoglobin (protein in charge of transporting oxygen from the lungs to the tissues and carbon dioxide from the tissues to the lungs, in addition to intervening in blood pH regulation).

An iron deficiency will therefore cause deficient haem synthesis, a lower production of haemoglobin and, as a consequence, a lower production of red blood cells (also called erythrocytes).

Depending on its severity, anaemia can be classified into chronic anaemia (low growth rate, apathy, cracked skin, rough hair and pale mucosae) or acute anaemia (laboured breathing and sudden death due to a lack of oxygen).

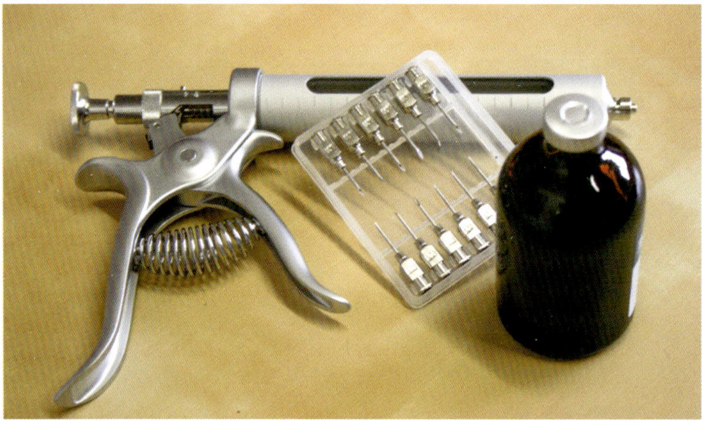

Figure 23 Instruments necessary to inject iron (gun, needles and iron).

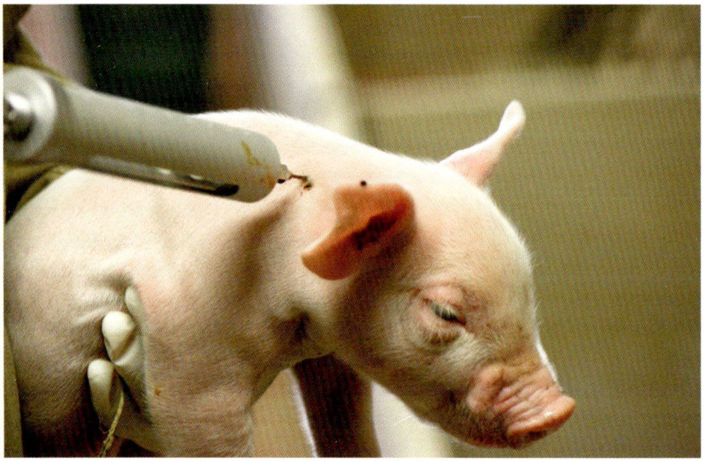

Figure 24 Iron administration to a piglet.

Piglets are born with very low iron reserves (approximately 50 mg) and have daily needs of 10-15 mg. They must therefore get supplemental iron from an external source in order not to rapidly consume their body reserves. There are several reasons why they require supplementary iron:

- Milk and colostrum have low iron levels and, unlike free-range pigs, piglets on intensive operations have no contact with the soil and do not consume iron from the environment through their rooting behaviour.
- The amount of iron accumulated in the piglet's tissues at birth is low.
- Piglets' rapid growth and the increase in their blood volume in their first few hours of life involves greater iron requirements. Piglets almost double their weight in their first week of life and have increased their weight by 5-6 times at four weeks old. The increase in their body and blood volume results in a rapid increase in iron requirements.

> A dose of 200 mg iron dextran or gleptoferron should be administered before piglets are three weeks old.

The administration of iron to sows by injection or through high iron levels in the feed has not given good results to increase iron levels in the body reserves of piglets. In some countries, iron is administered by oral route to piglets, but its level of absorption is low. Parenteral administration is more common and effective.

It is performed in the neck (never in the thighs to prevent injuries to the sciatic nerve that may cause lameness or reduce meat value due to abscesses) by inserting the gun or syringe perpendicular to the site (Fig. 24), with a thin and sharp needle and away from the spine so the bones or nerves are not affected. In order to avoid losses of the product after its inoculation, the skin should be stretched slightly to one side before the injection, so the orifice created in the skin does not coincide with that of the injection.

The needle should be replaced between litters to prevent the spread of infections.

Specific treatments

During this period, multiple treatments can be given to piglets. Some of them may be curative and others preventive, when the presence of a specific pathogen or pathological condition is certain. The most common treatments are listed next.

Vaccinations or preventive treatments (injectable or oral)

The vaccines or injectable antibiotic treatments administered during this period have a very specific objective: protecting piglets against specific pathogens and diseases. Maximum hygiene should be ensured during the procedure and administration guidelines should always be followed. Needles –in the case of intramuscular administration– or drench nozzles –in the case of oral administration– must be changed between litters. The treatments in this category include vaccinations against enzootic pneumonia, Glässer's disease or circovirus infections, as well as the administration of coccidiostatic drugs (toltrazuril) to prevent clinical signs caused by *Isospora suis.*

Inguinal hernia surgery

Occasionally, the inguinal canal, which is the duct containing the vas deferens and blood vessels irrigating the testicles, has a larger size than usual and makes it possible for the intestine to slip down into the scrotal sac, thereby creating a hernia. It is important to identify this problem before castration to avoid causing injuries to the intestine. Hernias sometimes become strangulated, which affects the intestine and causes intestinal transit disorders that may eventually lead to death of the animal.

To solve this problem, the piglet should be sedated and the procedure should be carried out as if it were a normal castration. However, it should ideally be performed at 3-4 weeks of age. The animal is placed with the abdomen facing upwards. The hernia is identified and the testicle is grasped with the fingers to elevate it as much as possible in order to palpate the inguinal canal. An incision is then made with a scalpel through the skin surrounding the inguinal canal, with care not to cause any injuries to the tunica that covers the testicle or to other structures, which could cause the herniated abdominal contents to come out. The tunica is pushed in to move the herniated contents back into the abdomen. Next, the structures are sutured as close as possible to the abdomen with a needle and nylon thread. The spermatic cord and sac are included in the suture and a double knot is made. The sac is then cut above the suture to remove the testicle and an antibiotic is applied on the suture (a broad-spectrum antibiotic should also be administered by injection). To complete the procedure, the skin is sutured and a topical disinfectant or healing agent is applied on the incision.

Castration

On some operations, the surgical removal of the testicles is performed on male pigs for slaughter. The purpose is to obtain meat products characterised by a fatty deposit and by the absence of boar taint, a consequence of the production of two natural substances that accumulate in fat tissues when males reach sexual maturity or puberty:

- Androsterone: anabolic steroid that is produced in the Leydig cells of the testicle.
- Indole: metabolite produced after tryptophan degradation in the distal colon. Its derivative is skatole.

Boar taint can be an offensive odour to some consumers, especially when cooking the meat or eating it.

PROCEDURE TO CASTRATE A PIGLET UNDER 6 DAYS OLD

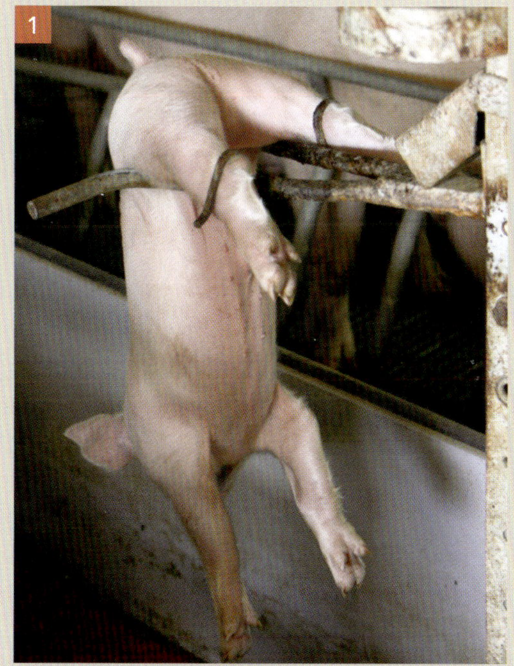

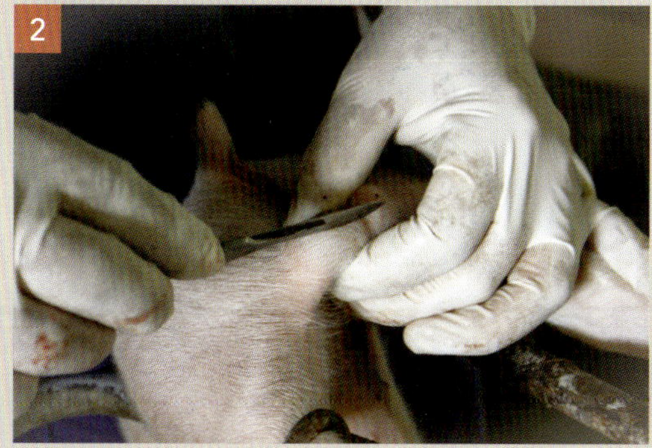

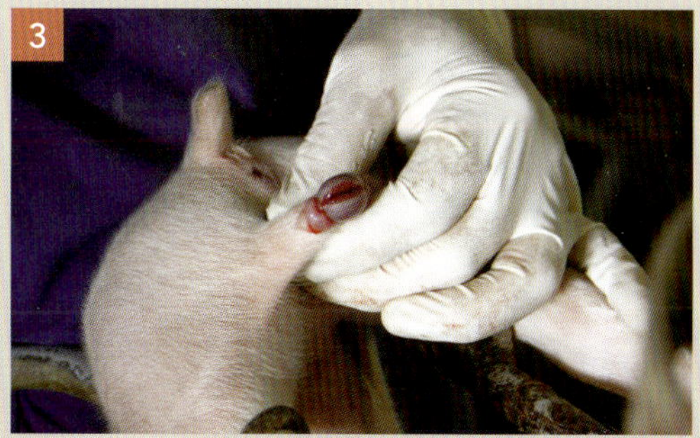

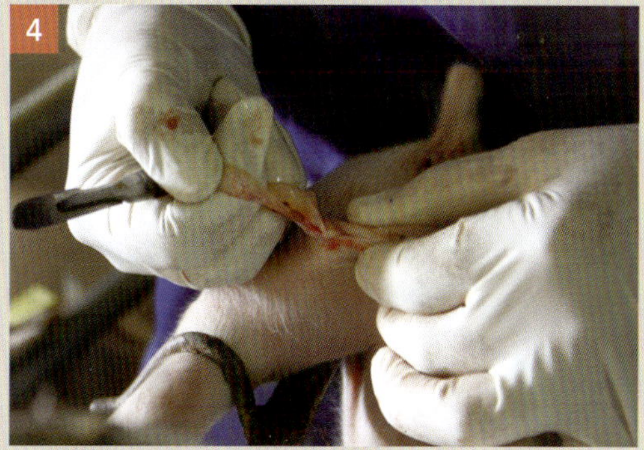

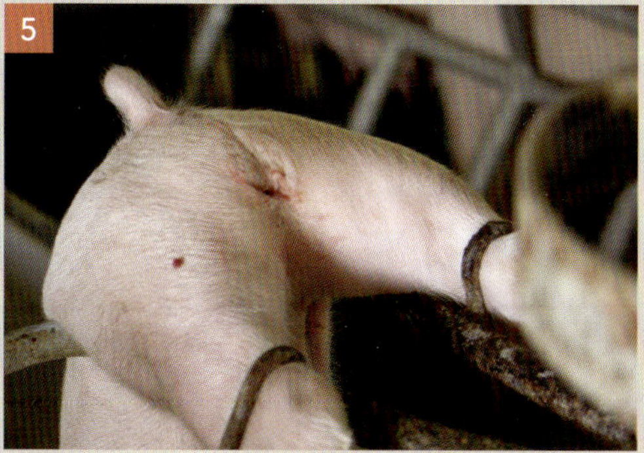

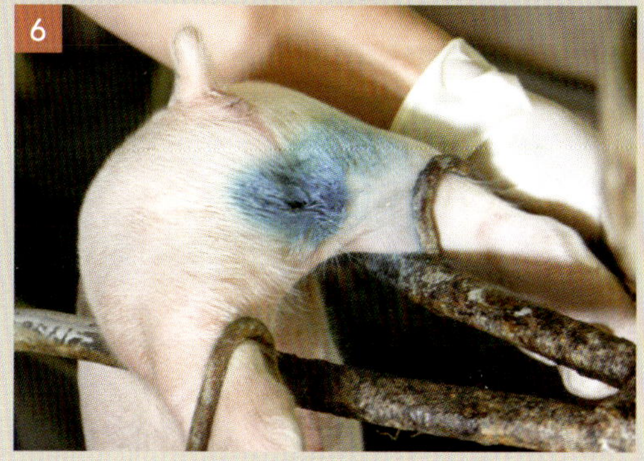

1. Piglet placed in a holder for castration.
2. Incision through the skin of the lower part of the scrotum.
3. Testicles protruding through the incision.
4. Cutting of the spermatic cord and blood vessels.
5. The castration process is complete, no sutures are made.
6. Application of a topical disinfectant.

Castration without anaesthesia is a very painful process for piglets. Some countries have consequently passed laws to prevent surgical castration with no anaesthesia.

The best time to castrate piglets is at 4-6 days of age. Piglets are easy to immobilise when they are small; they bleed less during the procedure and the protection obtained through their mother's colostrum is still effective. Piglets should not be castrated under 4 days of age, because the identification of inguinal hernias is more difficult and their testicles may sometimes have not descended.

To perform castration properly, a farm worker should hold the piglet by its lower limbs, with its head downwards (a holder may also be used to place the piglet in this position). Another worker must push the testicles up to expose them and make an incision through the skin of the lower part of the scrotum to allow for fluid drainage. Next, the testicles are pulled slightly and the spermatic cord and blood vessels are cut. A topical disinfectant is then applied on the wound, which is not sutured and will heal on its own. Maximum hygiene should be ensured during the process; the farm worker in charge of the task should wear disposable gloves and disinfect the area where the incision will be made.

Nevetheless, surgical castration without anaesthesia is a painful process characterised by high-pitched vocalisations, which indicate pain, and increased cortisol and corticotropin (ACTH) levels, which are a consequence of a stressful, painful and inflammatory process. In addition, postoperative pain may last for up to five days, during which the castrated animals show signs of pain in the affected area and are less active. It can also have negative effects on the animal's growth and immune system.

The European Union is looking for alternatives to avoid suffering in these animals. In the past few years, several injectable products causing immunocastration have appeared on the market, with a similar effect to that produced by the physical removal of the testicles.

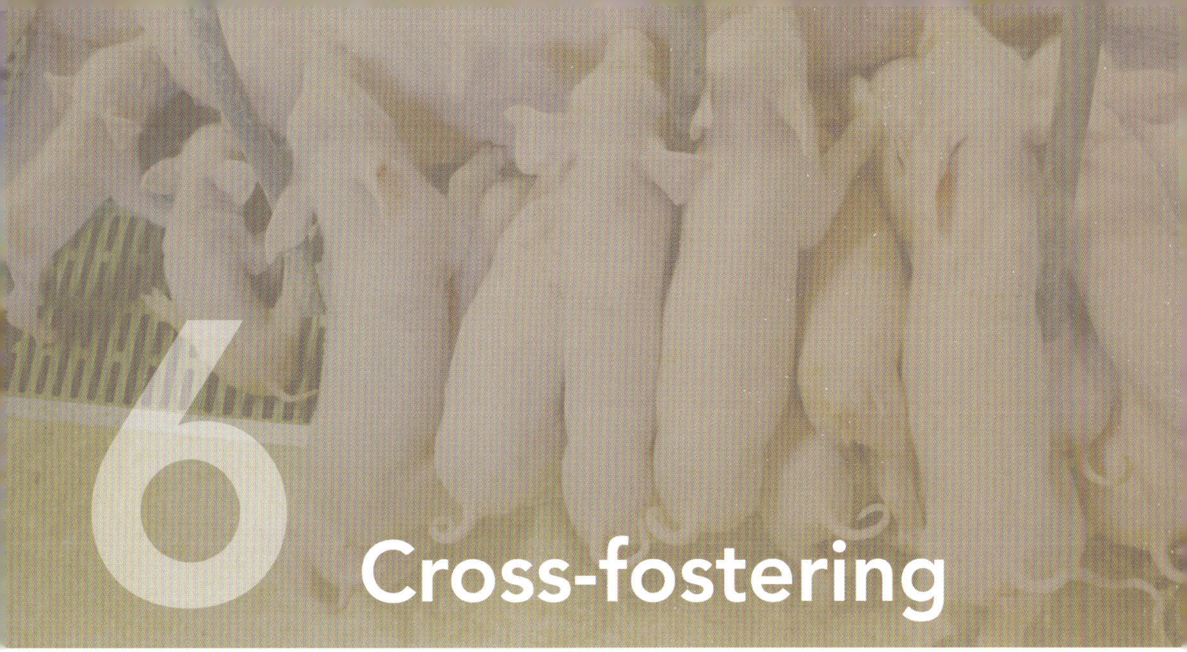

6 Cross-fostering

Introduction

Hyperprolific sow lines are capable of farrowing a large number of live piglets (up to 15-16 piglets per farrowing). Nevertheless, both the number of teats and the milk production of these sows are insufficient to nurse all the piglets that are born alive. It is thus essential to use a key practice in swine husbandry: **cross-fostering**. With this method, the productive potential of farms can reach more than 30 piglets per sow and year. This chapter provides detailed explanations of what this husbandry practice involves, of when it is necessary and of how it is performed.

Cross-fostering

When an operation weans an average of 13-14 piglets per sow and year, this does not mean that most of its sows reach this objective, but rather that most of them wean 12 piglets, while the best sows wean 13-14 piglets and a small percentage (nurse sows) raise two consecutive litters.

Cross-fostering is key on swine operations:

- **It improves the survival of small piglets in large litters.** These litters are characterised by greater weight variability at birth and difficulty to achieve an appropriate colostrum and milk intake.
- **It maximises the number of piglets produced per sow and year as well as their weight at birth.** The aim of cross-fostering is to ensure all piglets have access to a functional teat for the whole lactation period, thereby reducing preweaning mortality.

Example:

Farm with a batch of 40 sows: 32 sows wean 12 piglets on average, 4 sows wean 14 piglets on average, and the remaining 10 % (4 sows) are foster sows that nurse two consecutive litters of 12 piglets. An average number of 13.4 piglets are weaned per sow. The calculations are as follows:

- 12 piglets weaned from 32 sows: 32 x 12 = 384
- 14 piglets weaned from 4 sows: 4 x 14 = 56
- 24 piglets weaned from 4 nurse sows (two lactations of 12 piglets): 4 x 24 = 96
- 384 + 56 + 96 = 536 weaned piglets/ 40 sows = 13.4 piglets on average weaned per sow

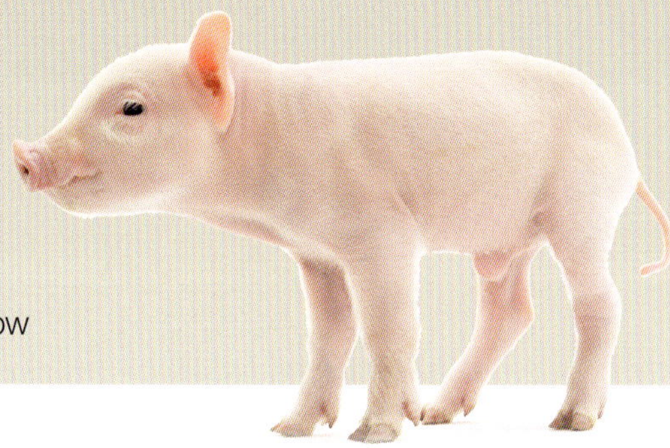

When to use cross-fostering

A swine operation should consider cross-fostering in the following cases:

- **Emergency fostering:** when a sow is sick or suffers from mastitis and cannot nurse her litter; to raise the piglets of a sow that died during lactation; or as a result of poor maternal behaviour (aggressive sow).
- **Cross-fostering due to a surplus of piglets or to make litters equal:** when there are more live piglets that functional teats and when there is significant variability in weight at birth in the litters.
- **Cross-fostering due to undernourished piglets** when the mother's milk production is insufficient (Fig. 1).

In all these cases, the best option is to choose a sow with good mothering abilities so she can foster a litter of piglets that are not hers. These sows that are given piglets from other sows are **foster or nurse sows**.

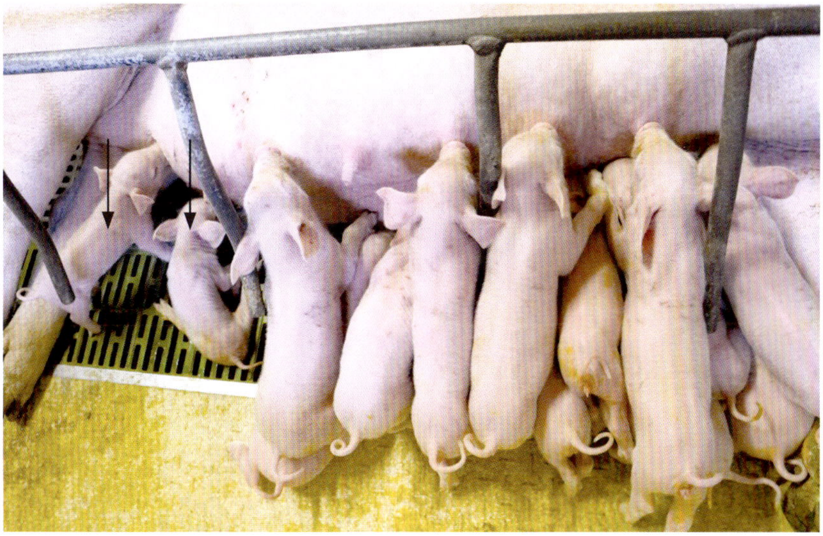

Figure 1 Small piglets (arrows) that should be transferred to a nurse sow.

Nurse sow

A nurse sow is a sow that, after having nursed her piglets completely (if her piglets are weaned) or partially (if they are transferred before the end of the lactation period to a sow that farrowed earlier), fosters a litter that is not hers.

Characteristics of nurse sows

These sows are chosen in each batch by looking for the characteristics of the "ideal sow". To do so, the aspects detailed next are taken into consideration.

The udder

The quality of the mammary glands is always a critical characteristic when it comes to selecting a nurse sow. A visual examination of the following should be carried out:

- **Number of teats and viability.** It is essential never to have more piglets than functioning teats on the sows. The mammary glands are thus examined to check for any injured teat, signs of mastitis or to ensure they are really functional.
- **Exposure of the teats.** Sometimes, the upper row of teats is too high (this usually occurs in old sows) or some teats of the lower row are not accessible to the piglets. If the mammary glands are very close to each other, access to all the teats is also compromised. In addition, it should also be borne in mind

that inguinal teats sometimes remain under the sow's leg and are not very accessible to the piglets.

- **Size and shape of the teats.** The chosen sow should preferably have long and thin teats, as this promotes nursing in the smallest and weakest piglets. Short teats make it difficult for piglets to nurse. For this reason, second or third-parity sows are usually used as nurse sows.

Sow's history

The sow's history should be checked in the farrowing unit records, as it will provide information about her previous farrowings and the number of piglets she was able to nurse properly. Sows that have farrowed more than three or four times should not be given more piglets than those they had in their previous lactation, even if their teats are in good condition.

Number of farrowings

As a general rule, the ideal nurse sow is a **second-parity** sow. The usual recommendation is to use first-parity sows to foster small piglets, as the morphology of their mammary glands is generally optimal (good exposure, many functional mammary glands and thin teats). However, gilts tend to have a poorer milk ejection reflex, which, together with the fact that piglets sometimes cannot suckle effectively, makes it more difficult for the latter to nurse. When a first-parity sow is used as a nurse sow, she should be given the strongest piglets in the batch in order to enhance her mammary development and optimise her milk production in this lactation and the following. Sows that are going to be culled should preferably not be used to nurse piglets that are too

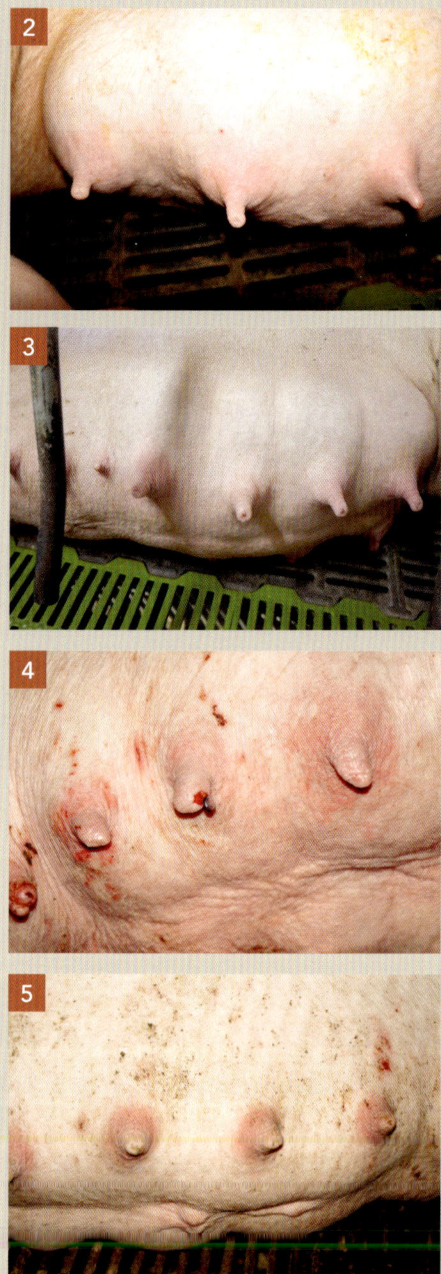

Figures 2 to 5 Different types of teats. The degree of difficulty with which the piglets will suckle depends on their morphology. The images are displayed according to suitability of the teats: they are thin and long in Figs. 2 and 3, short and thick in Figs. 4 and 5.

small to be weaned, as they are old sows with usually long and thick teats and a poorer milk production, or sows with a poorer history than average.

Maternal characteristics

The selected nurse sow should be quiet. A written or computer record of the sows with good mothering abilities should be kept so these can be used as nurse sows in future lactations.

In addition, it is important to ensure the sow has an optimal body condition and a good health status.

Cross-fostering process

Nurse sows can be selected and cross-fostering carried out from the day of farrowing to the time of weaning.

The usual cross-fostering processes are explained in detail next:

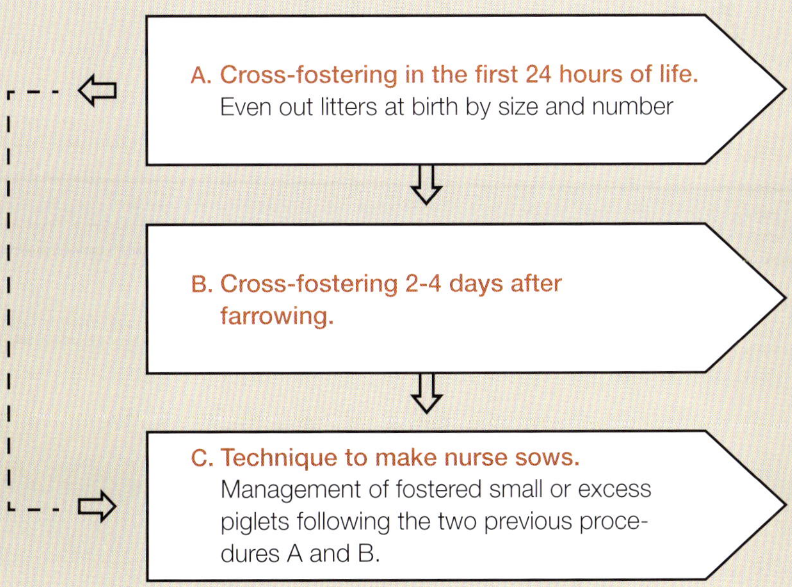

A. Cross-fostering in the first 24 hours of life

Due to the high prolificacy of sows, evening out litters after farrowing is the first step to achieve a successful start to the lactation period. Before moving any piglets from one sow to another, it is essential to make sure they have ingested a sufficient amount of colostrum from their mother. Once this has been ensured –especially in those litters where some piglets do not have an easy access to the udder (large litters, inaccessible or non-functional teats...)–, the earlier the piglets are moved, the better, as fights over the same teat will be avoided. It should be remembered that two piglets cannot nurse at the same teat.

Litters should be evened out between **12 and 24 hours postpartum**. The time at which the sows have farrowed should be taken into account. Ideally, farrowings should be monitored and their date as well as their start and end times should be recorded. One of the advantages of synchronising farrowings is that most of them will take place in the morning and litters can therefore be evened out in the afternoon. The choice of the time to perform this task depends on the work schedule on the operation. A possible schedule would be the following:

- Farrowings in the morning ⇨ evening out litters in the afternoon,
- farrowings in the afternoon ⇨ evening out litters the next morning,
- farrowings in the evening ⇨ evening out litters at the end of the next morning.

Bearing in mind the recommendations given on the next page, the best option to start with the cross-fostering procedures is to even out the litters in a batch by size and number.

A.1 Evening out litters by size

This is done so that all piglets in a litter start the lactation period with the same opportunities as the others and can reach their maximum growth potential. In order to even out litters, piglets can be divided into three categories: large, medium and small. To minimise the number of changes, the piglets that do not fit in the litter, that is, those that are in a minority, should be removed.

Recommendations

- Ideally, the piglets in a litter should be of a similar size: large, large and medium, medium, medium and small, small.
- **Small and large piglets should never be left in the same litter.**

Evening out litters successfully in the first 24 hours of life. Recommendations

- Litters should be evened out in the first 24 hours of life, after the piglets have consumed colostrum from their mother. It should be remembered that piglets start to select a teat a few hours after their birth and establish their hierarchy from the second or third day of life. Therefore, the later litters are evened out, the more the piglets will suffer in the process, as they will have got used to their hierarchy at the udder: new fights will take place, the sows will be more restless and the likelihood of them rejecting the fostered piglets will increase. To know whether a piglet has had enough colostrum, the best is to palpate its stomach to check whether it is filled.
- As few piglets as possible should be moved. Too many changes will stress the piglets and the sows.
- Piglet weighing more than 1.5 kg should not be moved before six hours after birth and those weighing less than 1.5 kg before 12 hours after birth. This is a way of ensuring they have had colostrum, as the heaviest piglets are also the most active.
- Sows can only nurse as many piglets as their number of functional teats.
- If newborn piglets are going to be fostered by a sow that has already been lactating for three days, it will be necessary to check whether her free teats are functioning prior to moving the piglets, as when mammary glands are not stimulated, they cease to produce milk after three days.
- The weakest and smallest piglets should be provided with the best conditions possible.
- When litters are very large (more piglets than functional teats in the batch): make nurse sows. Transfer the largest piglets with a filled stomach (Figs. 6 and 7) and dry umbilical cord to the sows that farrowed a week earlier (see *Technique to make nurse sows*, page 127).

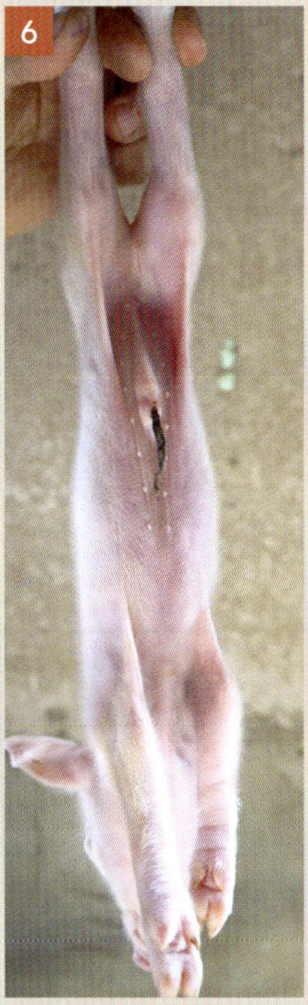

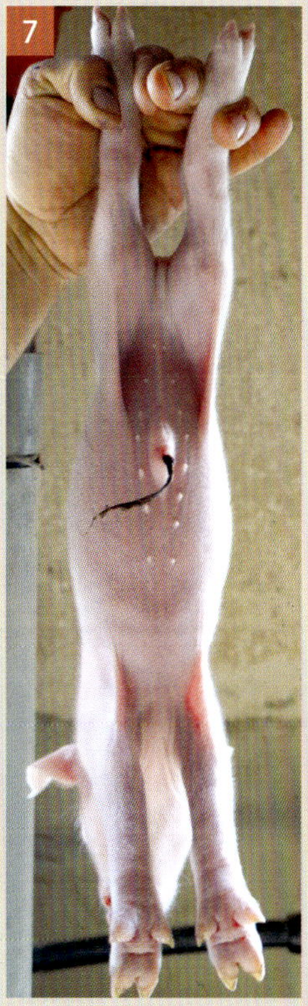

Figures 6 and 7 Difference between the aspect of a piglet with an empty stomach that has not yet ingested colostrum (Fig. 6), and that of a piglet with a stomach filled with colostrum (Fig. 7).

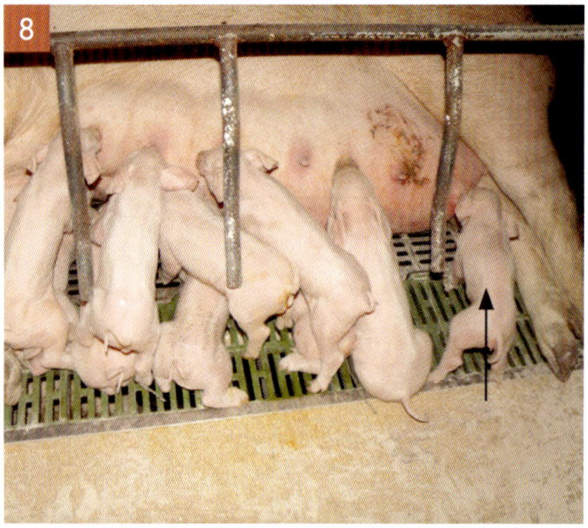

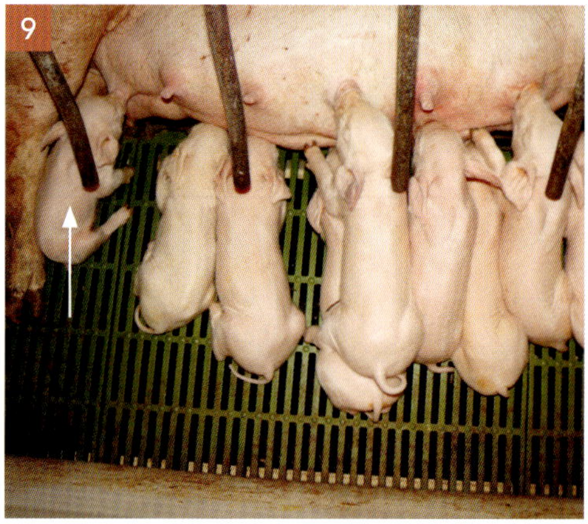

Figures 8 and 9 Litters from which the smallest piglets should be removed (arrows).

- On farms where most piglets are well developed at birth, it is preferable to remove the largest ones to make nurse sows and put the smallest and weakest piglets together to form a new litter.
- The current tendency is to leave the largest and strongest piglets with first-parity sows to promote the development of their mammary glands, and to use the best sows, which are usually second-parity sows, to nurse litters of smaller piglets.
- Once the small piglets are put together in the same litter, they should be provided with an additional energy source (natural or artificial colostrum).
- It is better to leave the smallest piglets with a sow with long, thin and well-exposed teats. If a sow with these characteristics has a high percentage of small piglets, it is best to leave them with her and to remove the largest piglets so they can be placed with another sow, and small piglets from other litters can be transferred to the first sow.

A.2 Evening out litters by number

The most recommended option is to even out litters by carefully assessing the quality and number of functional teats of each sow, so as to give them the exact number of piglets they can nurse. This process can be planned before farrowing by recording the number of piglets that can be left with the sow, so the cross-fostering process is carried out more easily (Fig. 10).

The litters should be checked up on 24 and 48 hours after they have been evened out, in order to look for piglets that cannot suckle properly and remove them to prepare new litters for nurse sows.

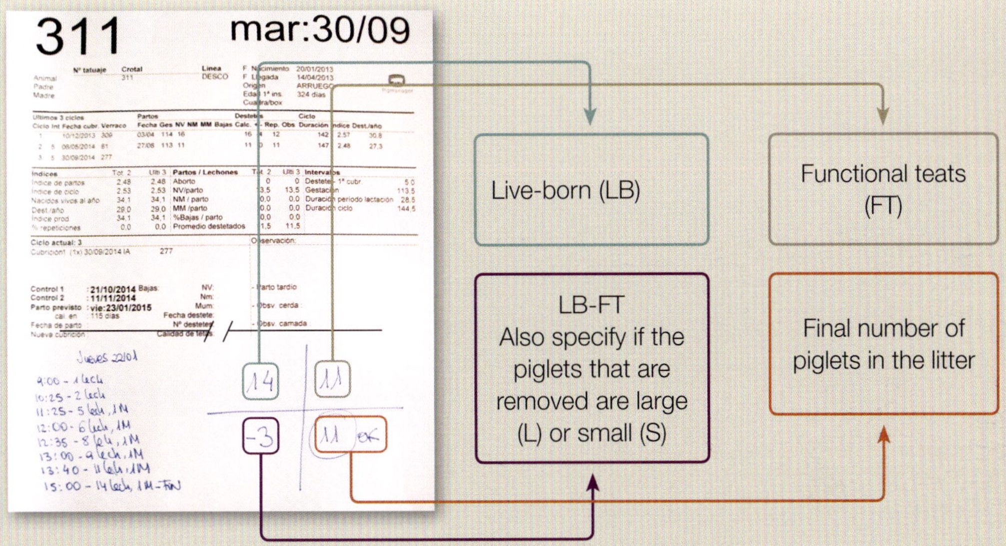

Figure 10 Farrowing unit record sheet with the information related to the cross-fostering process.

A.3 How to even out litters by size and number

Figure 11 shows an example of an imaginary situation in which eight sows from the same batch have farrowed on the same morning. The sows were monitored during farrowing and all the piglets have had sufficient colostrum. While the farrowing unit workers were monitoring the sows, they also wrote down all the relevant information on a record sheet or in a report:

- Characteristics of the teats: long and thin, short and thick...
- Number of functional teats.
- Number of piglets born alive.
- End time of the farrowing process. This last piece of information should be very clear and must be recorded to know when litters should be evened out.
- Based on these notes, the litters should be evened out by size and number on the afternoon of the same day. The objectives should be to optimise the number of functional teats and select the best sow for each type of piglet.

Once the piglets have been moved and a nurse sow has been made for the excess piglets (see *Technique to make nurse sows*, p. 127), it is necessary to check for any piglet doing poorly in the hours following the process. If such piglets are found, they should be placed with other sows (as explained in section B, p. 126) or put together to make a new litter for a nurse sow (section C, p. 127).

Step 1

Count the number of teats and piglets

- Total no. of teats: 97.
- Total no. of piglets born alive: 108.
- Calculation of the number of nurse sows required:
  Surplus piglets: 108-97=11. One nurse sow is enough.

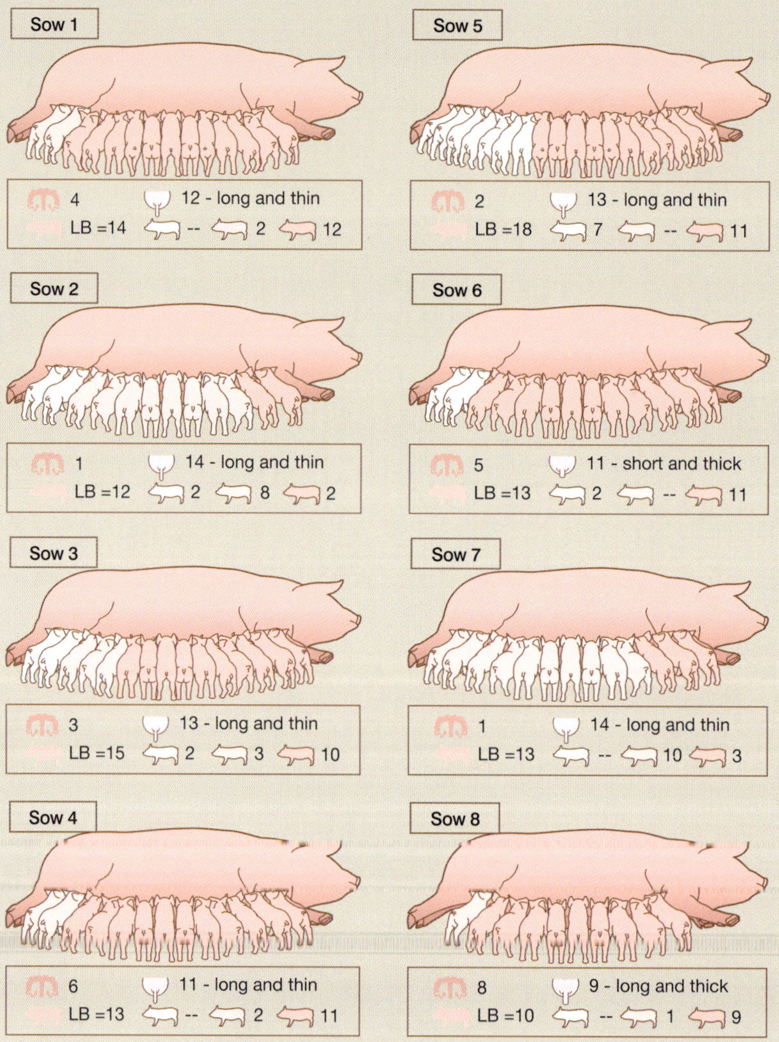

Figure 11 How to even out litters by size and number (steps 1 to 4).

Step 2

Select a nurse sow

Select piglets (if possible, medium or large) for a nurse sow and put all the small piglets together in a litter to give them to a nurse sow with a good history.

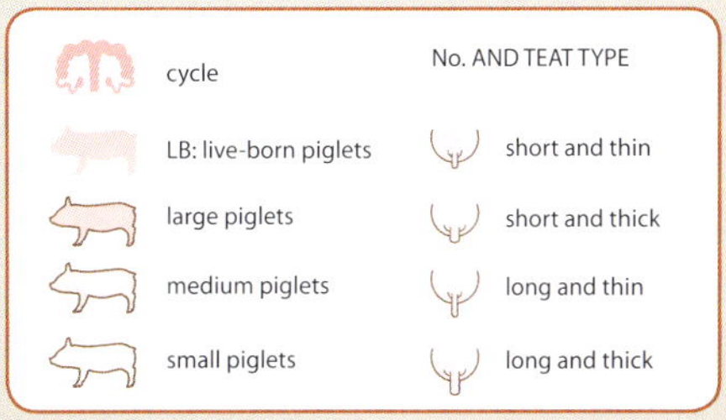

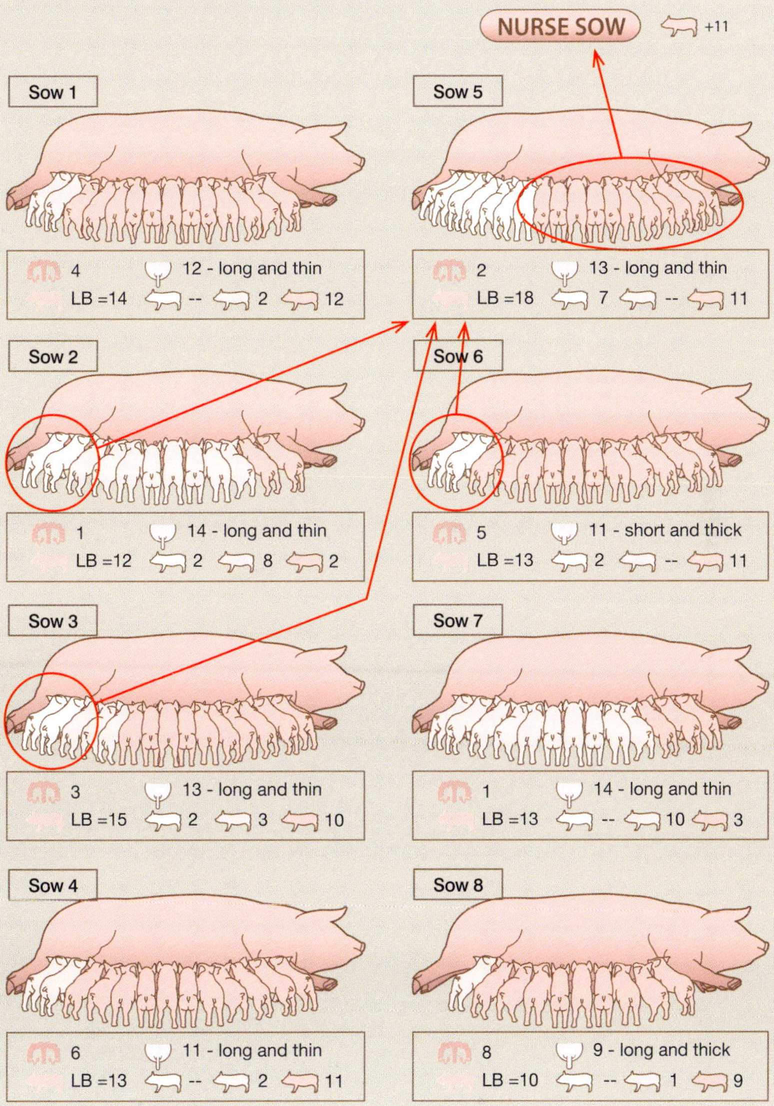

Step 3

Put all the small piglets together and even out the other litters

The weakest and smallest piglets have been put together in a litter and transferred to a sow with good characteristics. Her record sheet should indicate that she is fostering a litter of small piglets. Once the small piglets have been removed, the large and medium piglets can be left together without any problems. Nevertheless, the other litters should be evened out by size and number when possible, depending on the availability of functional teats and keeping changes to a minimum.

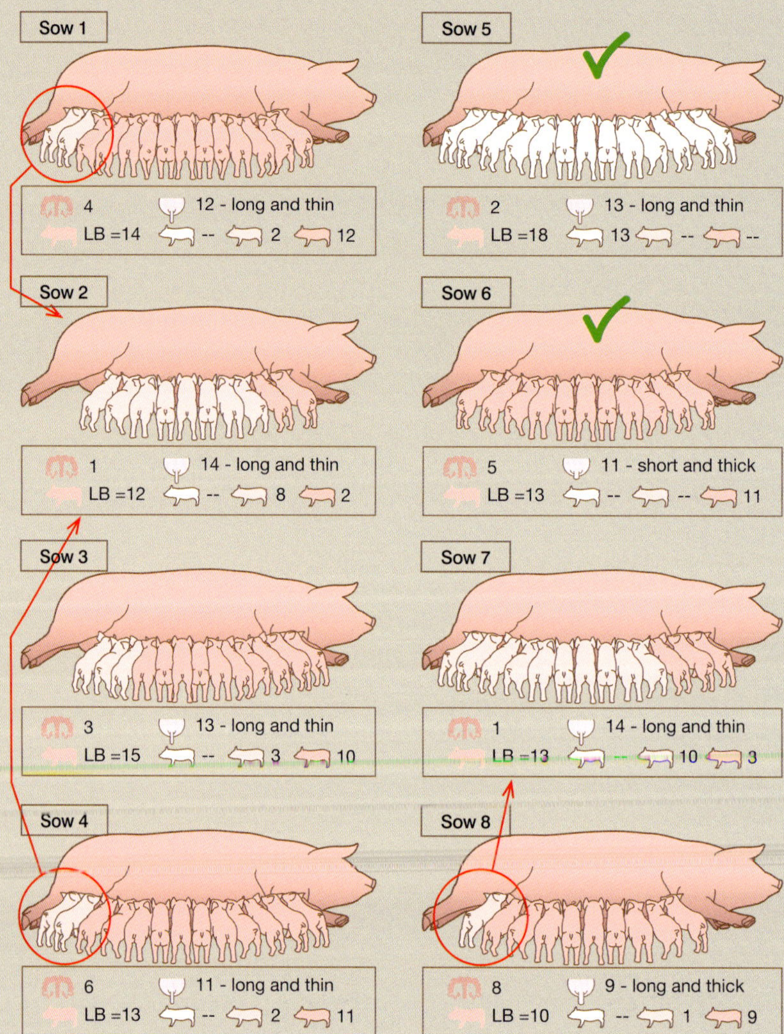

Step 4

Even out the rest of the litters

The litters have been optimised. Each sow has a number of piglets suited to her physiological capacities.

cycle		No. AND TEAT TYPE	
LB: live-born piglets		short and thin	
large piglets		short and thick	
medium piglets		long and thin	
small piglets		long and thick	

Sow 1

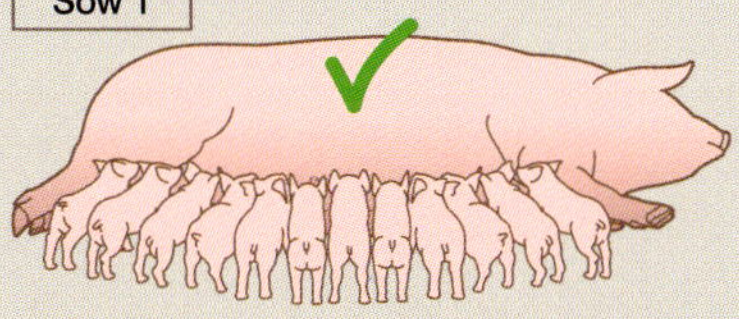

4 — 12 - long and thin
LB =14 -- -- 12

Sow 2

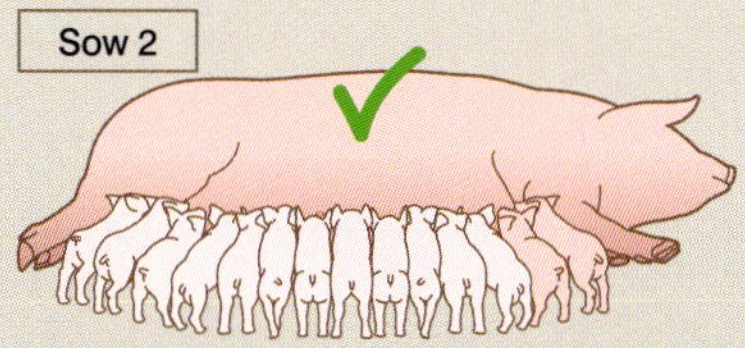

1 — 14 - long and thin
LB =12 -- 12 2

Sow 3

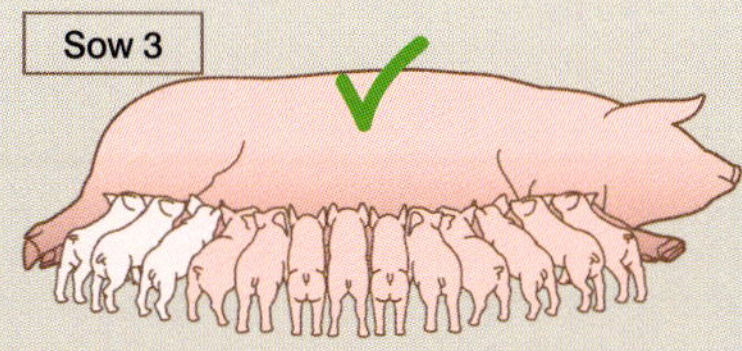

3 — 13 - long and thin
LB =15 -- 3 10

Sow 4

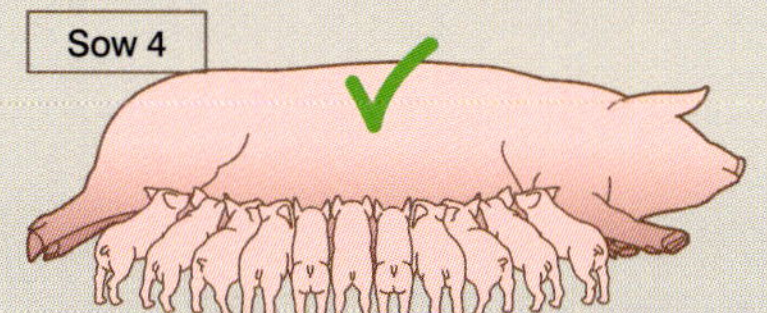

6 — 11 - long and thin
LB =13 -- -- 11

Sow 5

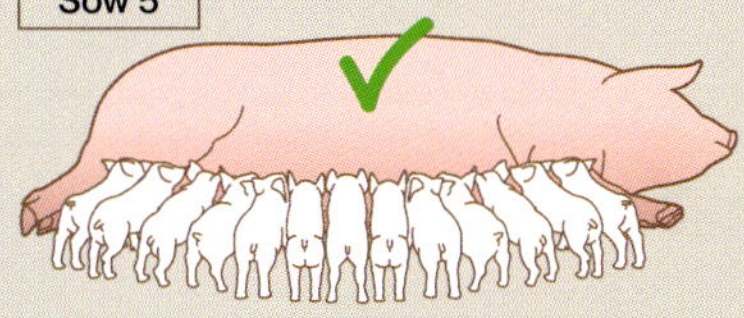

2 — 13 - long and thin
LB =18 13 -- --

Sow 6

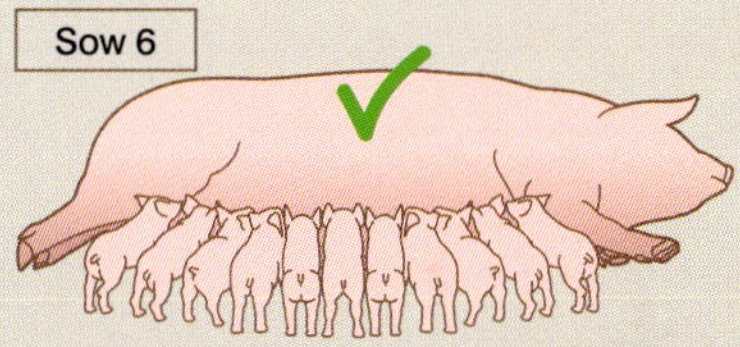

5 — 11 - short and thick
LB =13 -- -- 11

Sow 7

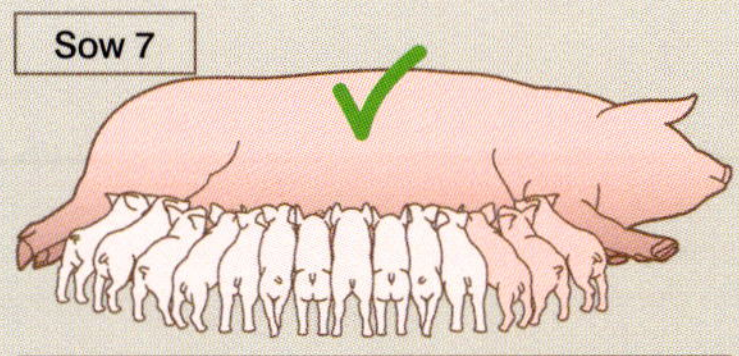

1 — 14 - long and thin
LB =13 -- 11 3

Sow 8

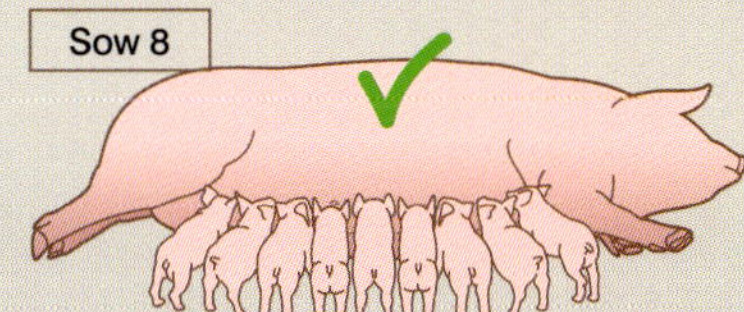

8 — 9 - long and thin
LB =10 -- -- 9

B. Cross-fostering 2-4 days after farrowing

Once the litters have been evened out at 12-24 hours of life, some piglets may only have access to a non-functional teat and must therefore be transferred to other sows. Since a mammary gland that is not stimulated will cease to produce milk after approximately three days, these piglets should be regrouped in the first three days of lactation.

The better litters are evened out, the fewer changes will be required subsequently. Moreover, piglets with a delayed growth should be identified rapidly to be transferred to another sow so they do not die of starvation. To do so, it is important to check for any thin and depressed piglets daily and to ensure their stomach is filled with milk (Figs. 12 and 13). Another functional teat must be found for these piglets, which should also be provided with energy supplements after they have been moved again.

The problem of this technique is that there is a risk of injuries and fights between the piglets that were already in the litter and the fostered piglets, as cross-fostering takes place when the hierarchy in the litter has already been established.

There are three options to solve this problem:

a) **Redistributing the piglets.** This practice is based on the fact that non-stimulated mammary glands stop producing milk after three days. This way:
   - It is possible to use the sows that were last to farrow in the batch (these are usually the least prolific) to even out their litters with the excess piglets.
   - Another option is to replace those sick piglets that have died (due to streptococcal infections, splay leg, or because they were born too weak to nurse effectively and stimulate milk let-down…) by other piglets.
   - This can also be done in case of deaths due to crushing, provided the sow shows good mothering abilities.

b) **Transferring piglets to a nurse sow.** If there are small piglets that cannot be transferred to a sow with free teats, a "nurse sow" should be made (as explained in the section *Technique to make nurse sows*, page 127).

c) **Swapping piglets across litters.** For very prolific genetic lines, some authors recommend removing the smallest piglets of each litter to give them to the best sow in each room. The strongest piglets of this sow will be placed with the other mothers, depending on how many piglets have been removed from each of them. Piglets with a delayed growth should be marked with a spray so they are identified and can be placed with a nurse sow if their condition does not improve.

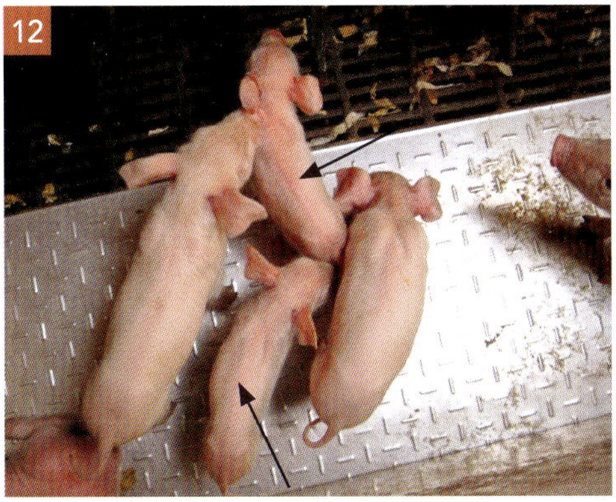

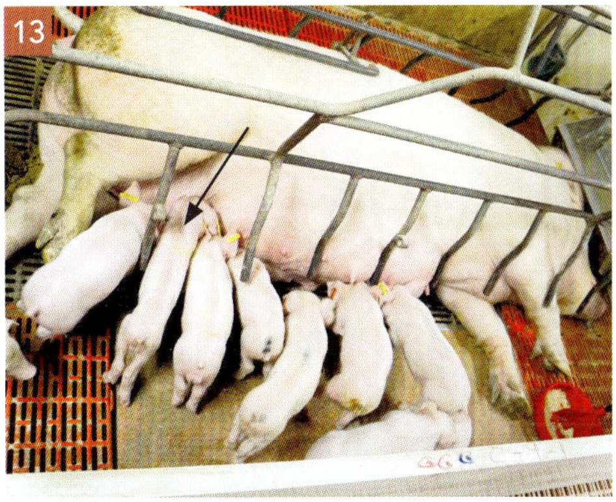

Figures 12 and 13 Small piglets can be observed in both images (arrows), as their spine is apparent (which indicates a low weight and starvation).

With this procedure, about 70 % of piglets recover, which avoids making more nurse sows.

When cross-fostering is practised, it is essential not to transfer:

- Piglets from litters with diarrhoea to healthy litters, as there is a risk of transmission.
- Small piglets about to be weaned to younger litters.
- Piglets of several days of age to a newly-farrowed sow, as her colostrum should be reserved to the piglets of her own litter.

> Piglets with a good growth after 3-4 days of life will end the lactation period successfully. However, it is very important to combine all these techniques (evening out litters, transferring piglets from one sow to another and making nurse sows).

C. Technique to make nurse sows

As previously explained, a nurse sow is a sow that fosters a litter that is not hers, after having nursed her litter completely or partially (page 115). It is very important to know how to choose calm sows with good mothering abilities. The fostered litter should have one piglet less than the litter the sow was previously nursing.

The **fostered piglets** will come from litters with too many piglets born alive, small or undernourished piglets, or from litters of sows that cannot nurse (death, diseases, physical problem or lack of milk production...).

> Weaning at 28 days of age and weekly batch farrowing offer greater flexibility to make nurse sows, as they do not require piglets to be weaned under 21 days of age.

There are two main techniques to make nurse sows, which are commonly called **"shunt fostering"**:

1. Shunt fostering by moving piglets.
2. Shunt fostering by moving sows.

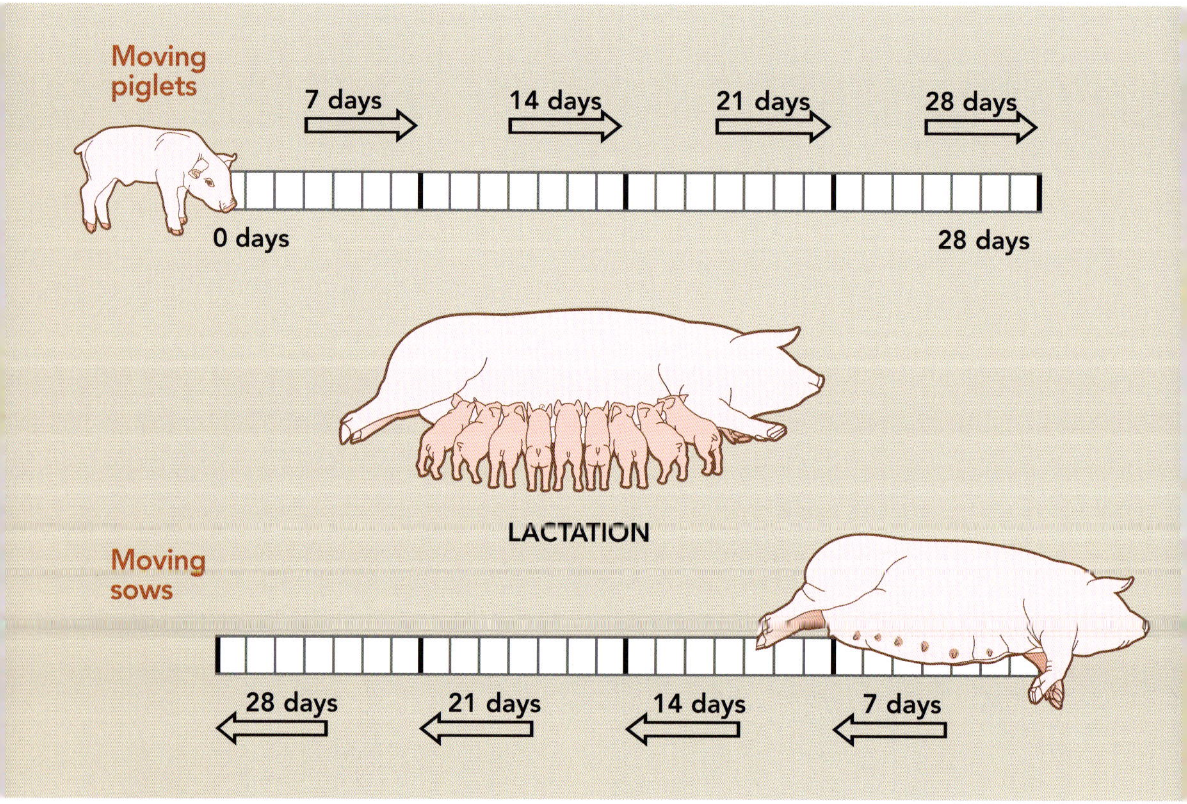

Figure 14 Representation of the two shunt fostering techniques.

C.1 Shunt fostering by moving piglets

The technique involves weaning piglets with an appropriate weight from a sow at an advanced stage of lactation (21-28 days) so she can foster the piglets of a sow from the previous batch, and so on. This process becomes clear with the following examples.

As the piglets are transferred to a sow at a more advanced stage of lactation, it is best to choose large individuals so they are of a similar size to those of the new litter, and can be weaned at a similar weight despite being younger.

Piglets should never be moved to a younger litter, as it can destabilise the health balance of the farm, since they will have been in contact with more microorganisms.

Example

How to make nurse sows by moving piglets up the age range

In the example, there are four rooms (each room corresponds to a batch), each with 20 sows. The sows are grouped in the different rooms according to how far into lactation they are. Piglets with a delayed growth start to appear on the next Monday on the operation (Fig. 15).

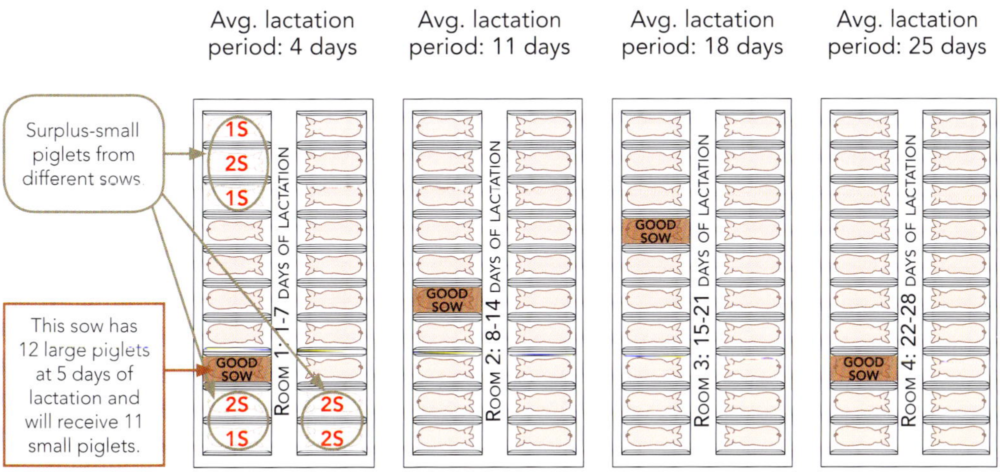

Figure 15 The 11 small piglets (S) are placed with a good sow.

Step 1

- The best option is to look for a good sow to nurse any surplus or small piglets in the batch (the number of small piglets is indicated with the letter "S", excess piglets are indicated with the letter "E"). If possible, it should also be one of the first sows to have farrowed in the batch. This way, the piglets that need to be transferred to the next batch are larger and the size difference with the piglets of the sow in the other batch will be smaller.
- The number of piglets to be fostered by the nurse sow should **never** be greater than the number of piglets she was nursing. In the example, the sow at 5 days of lactation had 12 piglets and is going to foster 11.

Step 2

Nurse sows should be chosen in the other batches and their piglets should be moved up the age range. The piglets of the sow in the most advanced batch are weaned so she can foster the other ones (Fig. 16). According to the example, the 5-day-old piglets will be fostered by a sow at 11 days of lactation, the 11-day-old piglets will be fostered by a sow at 18 days of lactation, and the 18-day-old piglets will be fostered by a sow at 25 days of lactation. The piglets of this sow will be weaned at 25 days of age and those she will foster will be weaned on the next Thursday at 21 days of age (18 + 3 days for the sow to complete the lactation period –from Monday to Thursday–).

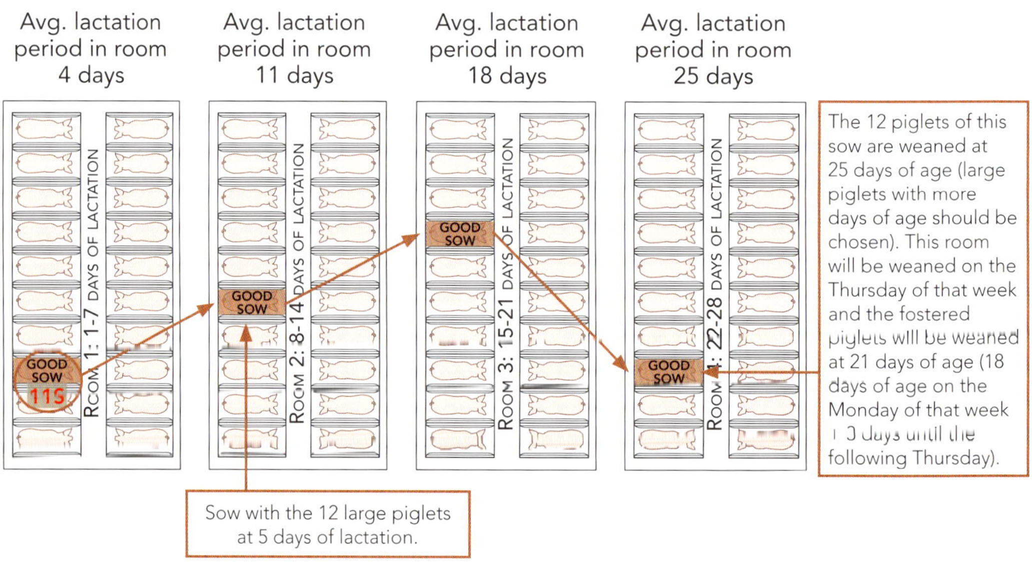

Figure 16 Moving litters to good nurse sows from more advanced batches. The good sow in room 1 receives 11 piglets with delayed growth and her 12 large piglets are transferred to the good sow in room 2.

Example with surplus piglets at birth

The example is similar if the first nurse sow is made with surplus piglets, the only difference being that the average time in lactation of the piglets in each batch will be lower. It is best to choose a sow with a strong litter from the same batch to minimise the size difference between the piglets that are moved up the age range.

The **advantage** of moving litters up the age range is that the farrowing target and the interval between farrowings on the operation are maintained, as it is not necessary to prolong the lactation period of the nurse sow, since all sows are weaned with the rest of their batch.

The **disadvantage** is that more litters are weaned earlier. Weaning will take place at about 21 days of age on farms with weekly batch farrowing that have enough room in the farrowing units to wean at four weeks of age. However, with batch farrowing every two or more weeks, or when piglets are weaned at three weeks of age, the piglets weaned from the last nurse sow are too young and small. For these reasons, on operations where prolificacy is very high, some farrowing places should be left empty to combine this technique with that of moving sows. This way, it is possible to avoid weaning many young piglets, for which adaptation to the transition phase will be more difficult.

C.2 Shunt fostering by moving sows

They key to this technique is to have **extra places** in the farrowing room. To create these places, the service target for each batch should be reduced. The recommendation is to reduce it by 10 % so extra places are available when the sows are moved to the farrowing unit. Another option is to design the farrowing unit with 10-20 % additional places. In order to use this technique, the weekly breeding target should not be exceeded and the farrowing rooms should only be filled with sows from the same batch, leaving extra places empty instead of using them for sows from the next batch.

The technique involves placing surplus piglets with a sow of the same batch that has farrowed a strong litter. This sow's piglets will be fostered by a sow with more days of lactation **which is moved to one of the extra places**. Ideally, there should be an interval of approximately seven days of lactation between the nurse sows from the different batches. The piglets of the sow at the most advanced stage of lactation and the largest piglets are weaned.

The sows that are going to be used as nurse sows and left in the farrowing unit can be chosen on the weaning day.

Example 1

Procedure with excess piglets

Let us take the example of an operation with 20 farrowing places for each batch. Piglets are weaned at 4 weeks of age and the farrowing target is 18 sows per week, 20-2 (10 %). This way, two places can be left empty. In this example, there is one single empty place (Fig. 17). The procedure would be the same with two empty places.

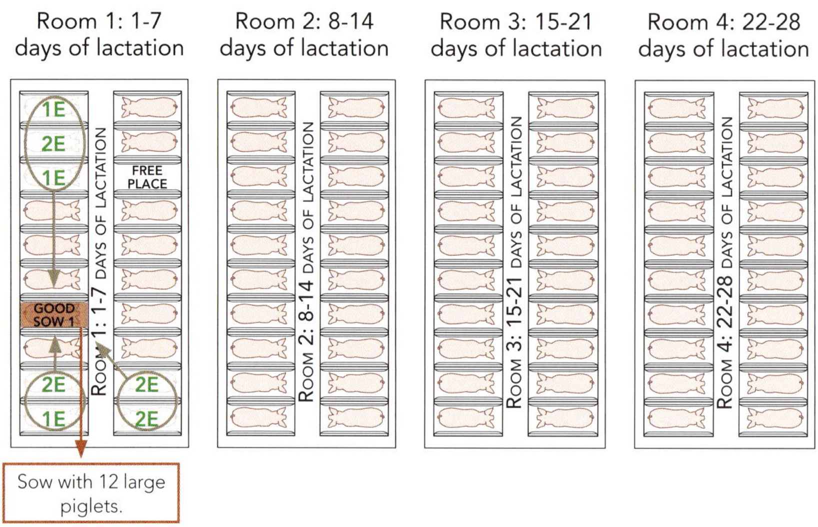

Figure 17 Example of shunt fostering by moving sows due to an excess of piglets.

Step 1

The first step is the same as with the previous technique: selecting a good sow to foster the surplus piglets of the batch.

Step 2

Selecting a good sow from another batch that will be moved to the empty place to foster the litter from the other sow. There are different options:

Option 1. Lactations prolonged by a week

The first place will be occupied by a sow from a more advanced batch that farrowed approximately seven days earlier. The empty place left by the sow will in turn be occupied by a sow from the next batch that farrowed seven days earlier, and so on. In this case, the sows are moved from one farrowing room to the previous room, as indicated in Figure 18.

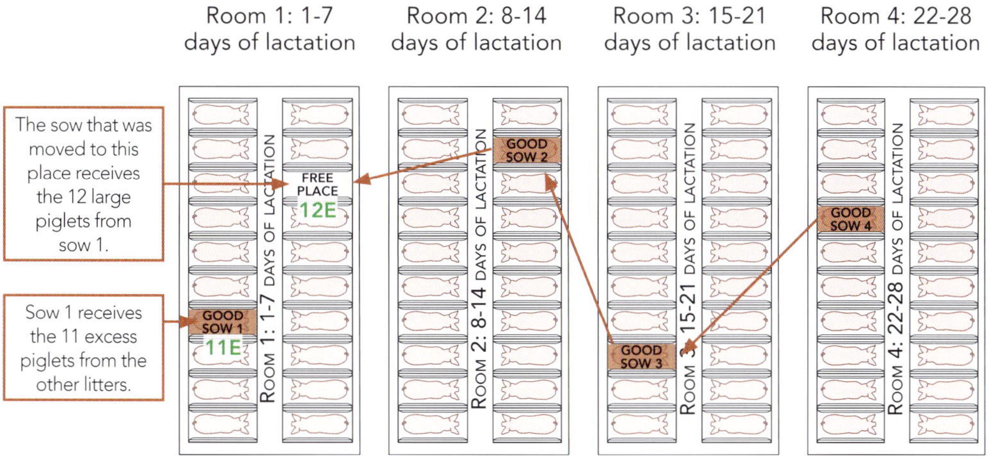

Figure 18 Representation of how the sows are moved to occupy the free places and foster piglets.

The process is as follows: sow 1 fosters the excess piglets of the batch. Sow 2 occupies the empty place in the first room, sow 3 the place left empty by sow 2 and sow 4 that left empty by sow 3. The piglets of sow 4 are weaned or remain in the farrowing unit in the same place, but without their mother. In this case, the nurse sows are weaned at 28 + 7= 35 days of lactation, as weaning is delayed by seven days for all of them (Fig. 19).

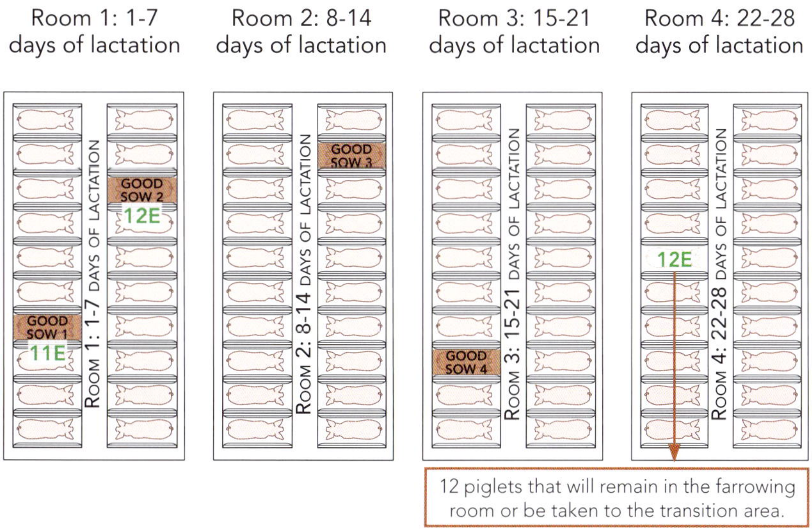

Figure 19 Location of the nurse sows after moving them to occupy the free places.

Option 2. Lactations prolonged by more than a week

This case may be common on farms with two-weekly batch farrowing, where the sows in a room have farrowed 14 days earlier than those in the next batch (the sows are weaned at 21 days + 14 = 35 days of lactation).

The changes with this option are more sudden: from room 4 to room 2 and from room 2 to room 1. Sow 3 is weaned at 42 days of lactation (28 days + 14) and sow 2 at 35 (28 + 7). With option 1, the lactation period is prolonged by 7 days for 3 sows and with option 2, it is prolonged by 14 days for 1 sow and by 7 days for the other. The average number of days of lactation is therefore the same with both options (21 days), option 1: 7 x 3; option 2: 14 + 7; Figs. 20 and 21.

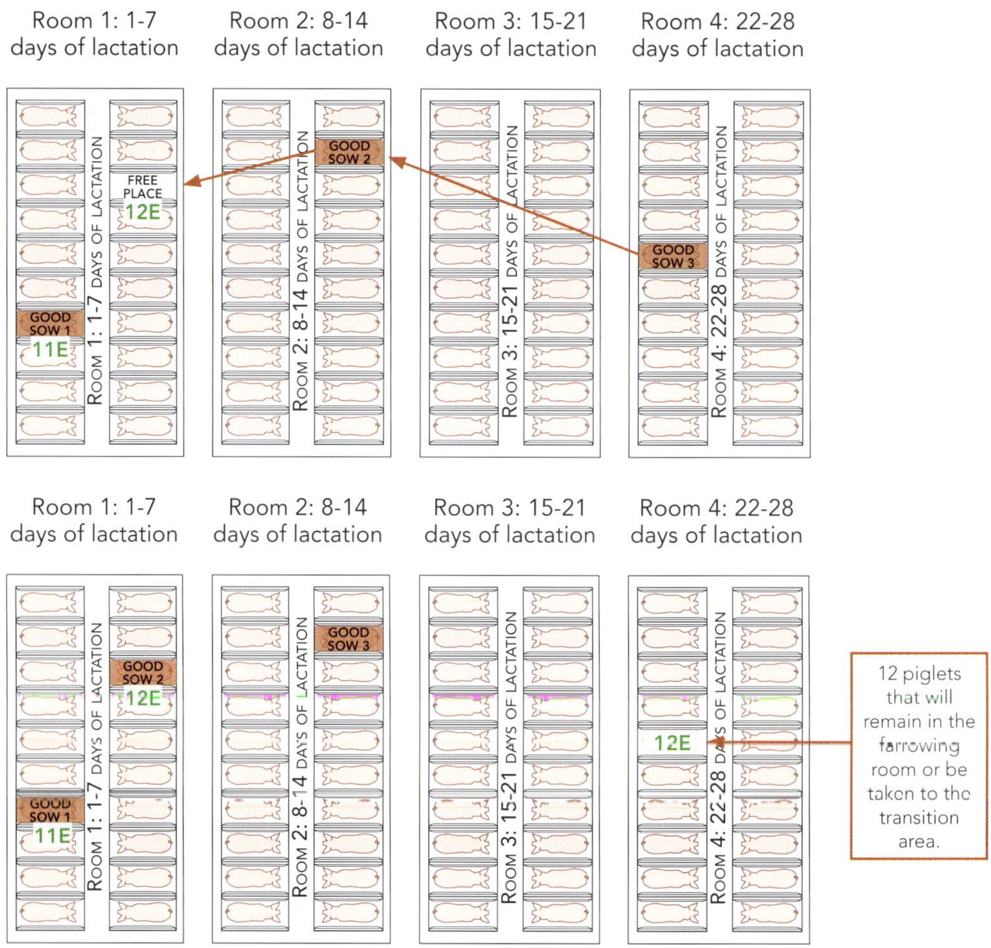

Figures 20 and 21 Occupation of the free places by the nurse sows (Fig. 20). Final result of the fostering procedures (Fig. 21).

Option 3

The third option would be to move one sow only, but it is very risky since the age and size difference between the piglets is considerable in this case.

Example 2

How to take advantage of the places that become available during lactation

Nurse sows can occupy the places of the sows to be culled (due to disease, agalactia, etc., or sows that have reached the end of their productive life), if the latter are sent earlier to slaughter (Fig. 22).

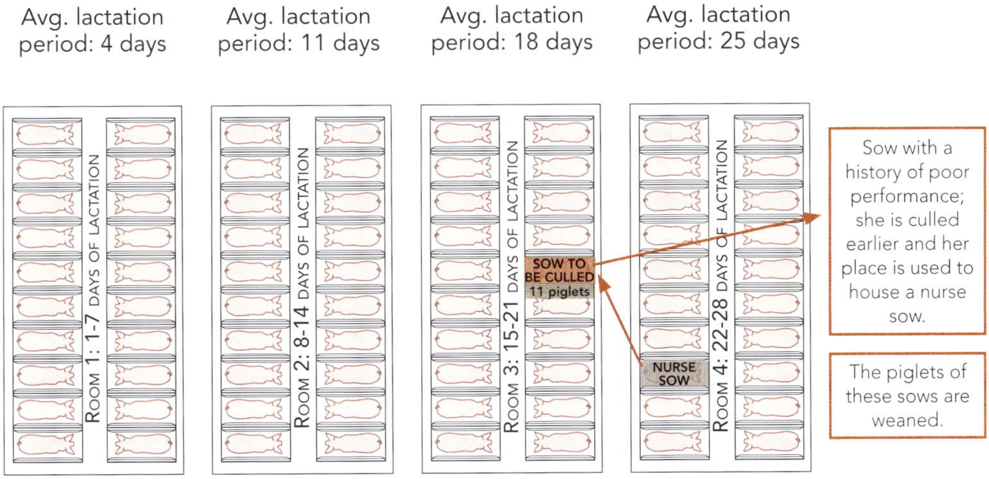

Figure 22 How to make nurse sows by taking advantage of the places that become available during lactation.

Example 3

When to use gilts as nurse sows

When making nurse sows by prolonging their lactation, first-parity sows can be used to favour their uterine involution. The days lost due to a longer lactation will be compensated for with a greater prolificacy in the next farrowing and a better weaning-to-fertile-service interval. For this to occur, the sow's body condition must be appropriate.

On farms where farrowing units are prepared to wean piglets at 21 days of age, it is interesting to make nurse sows by using the system with which a gilt's lactation is prolonged by a week (Figs. 23-25).

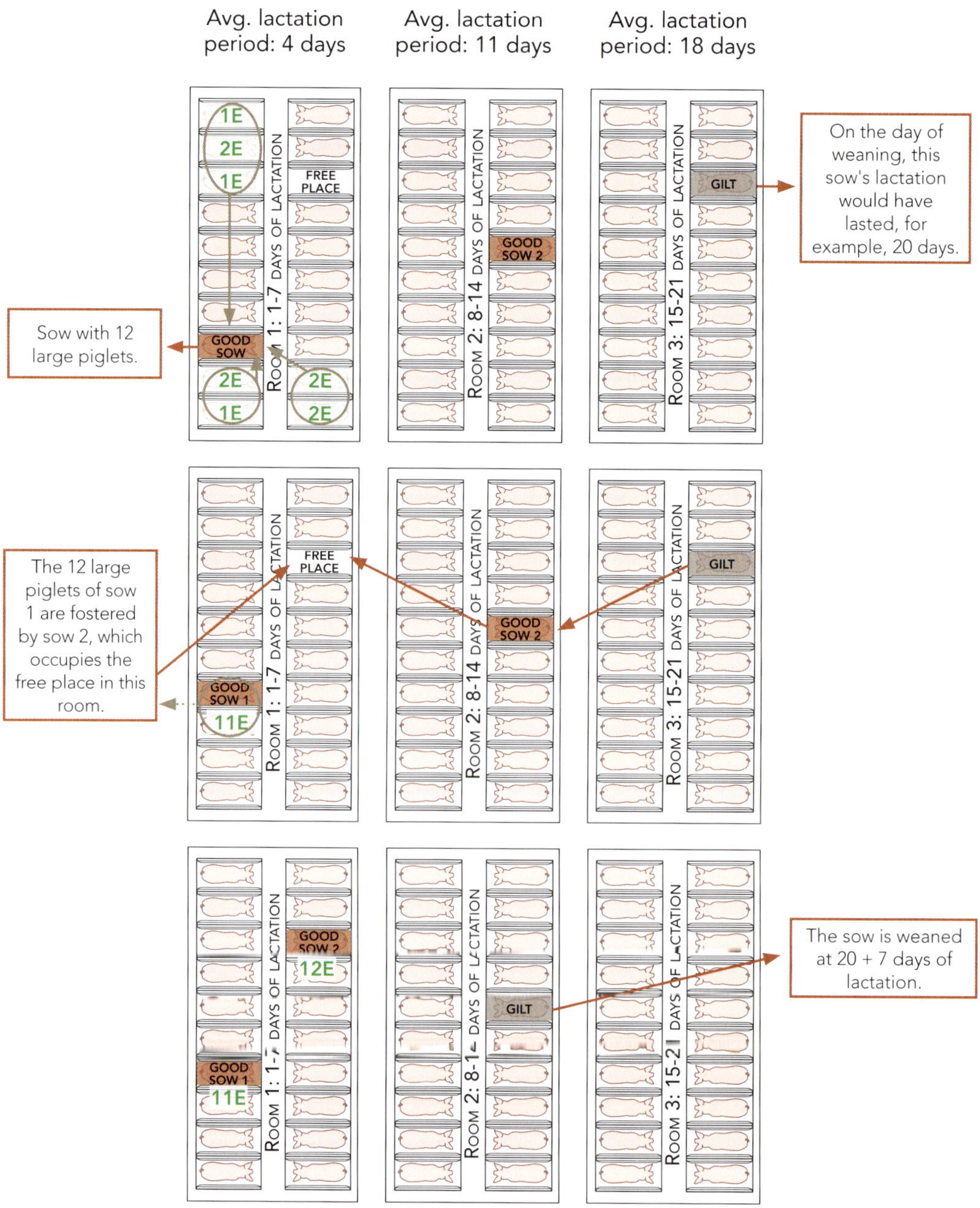

Figures 23 to 25 How to use first-parity sows as nurse sows.

The main **advantage** of this technique is that when the lactation period of nurse sows is prolonged, it is possible to move them to a batch with much younger piglets. Nonetheless, very sudden changes may cause them to reject their new litter as they will notice a decrease in the piglets' milk intake; they may even come in heat in the farrowing house. In addition, the litters are kept with their batch and most of the piglets are weaned at the standard age, except those of the last sow, which may be weaned a few days earlier.

Any empty places in the farrowing unit should be taken advantage of to use this system. However, the best option for an optimal use of the places in a farrowing unit is to **combine the two systems**, as the increase in the farrowing interval of nurse sows when the second technique is applied is compensated for by an increased productive performance on the farm, since mortality is reduced and more piglets are weaned.

Advantages and disadvantages of cross-fostering

Cross-fostering systems have, as previously explained for each technique, both advantages and disadvantages. These are summarised in Table 1 so they can be compared.

SYSTEMS	Advantages	Disadvantages
Cross-fostering (in general)	• Increased productive performance. • Low birth-to-weaning mortality. • High weaning weight.	• Cross-fostering requires a specialised workforce and time.
Shunt fostering by moving piglets	• The farrowing target and interval are maintained.	• Piglets moved from one room to another. • Age at weaning is reduced for some piglets.
Shunt fostering by moving sows	• Management is more convenient. It is easier to move sows rather than piglets from one room to another. • Fostered piglets are weaned with their batch.	• More places needed in the farrowing unit. • The farrowing interval is longer, as the lactation period of the nurse sows is increased.

Table 1 Advantages and disadvantages of the different fostering systems.

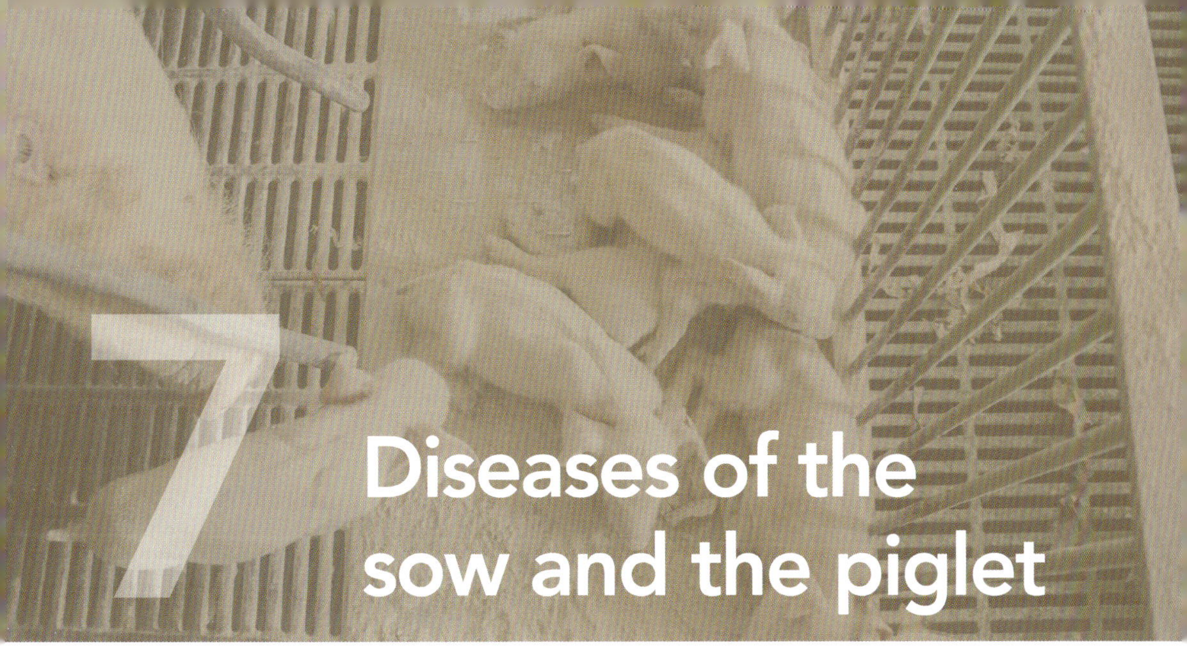

7 Diseases of the sow and the piglet

Introduction

In terms of health, the objective during the lactation period is to produce a flow of piglets with a high health status and a low mortality rate, since this has a direct impact on the number of weaned piglets per sow and per farrowing, as well as on their subsequent growth during the fattening period.

This chapter reviews the main diseases that affect sows and piglets during lactation according to their causes and severity, and the main prevention measures and programmes.

Main diseases of sows during the lactation period

Postpartum dysgalactia syndrome (PDS), metritis and mastitis are frequently observed in the first days of lactation. Postpartum dysgalactia syndrome is characterised by a reduction in milk production and fever of variable intensity. These signs may be accompanied by vaginal discharge and, on many occasions, by generalised apathy. Metritis appears in the form of purulent secretions through the vagina. Mastitis is the acute or chronic inflammation of one or more of the sow's mammary glands.

Gastrointestinal diseases

Gatrointestinal diseases are one of the main causes of mortality in sows during lactation. The diseases most commonly observed in farrowing units are described next.

Oesophageal and gastric ulcers

There are several types of ulcers depending on the exact location where they develop in the stomach. The most frequent are those of the aglandular area (Fig. 1), which surrounds the entrance of the oesophagus into the stomach. Those that affect the glandular area are often associated with systemic diseases.

Ulceration of the oesophageal part of the stomach is the most common type of gastric ulcer. It may trigger sudden death due to acute intragastric haemorrhage (Fig. 2) or become chronic. The animals suffering from gastric ulcers are apathetic and pale due to the internal bleeding. In most cases, the prognosis is death of the affected animal.

The aetiology of gastric ulcers is very varied with different risk factors, many of them associated with the physical presentation of the feed:

- Finely ground particles of raw ingredient with a size below 500 microns. Fine grinding improves feed digestibility but also increases the risk of ulcers.
- A lack of size homogeneity in the particles, due to an inappropriate grinding with the presence of very thin particles, is a predisposing factor.
- Grain processed with a hammermill tends to cause more ulcers than when it is processed with a roller mill.
- Ulcers are more frequent with pelleted feed than with mash feed.
- Oats and barley have a lower ulcerogenic effect than corn and wheat.
- Selenium and vitamin E deficiencies are associated with a greater incidence of gastric ulcers.
- Fasting increases the incidence of ulcers.
- Some degree of seasonality is observed. Ulcers appear more frequently in the summer months.
- The presence of concomitant diseases is another predisposing factor.
- The appearance of ulcers increases as the farrowing date approaches.
- There is some genetic predisposition.
- Infection by *Ascaris* also seems to be a predisposing factor.

Clostridial diseases

Clostridium novyi is a bacterium naturally found in the intestine of pigs. In certain situations of stress, it produces spores that germinate, which gives rise to toxins that usually cause death due to a hyperacute state of toxaemia, known as **sudden death syndrome in sows**.

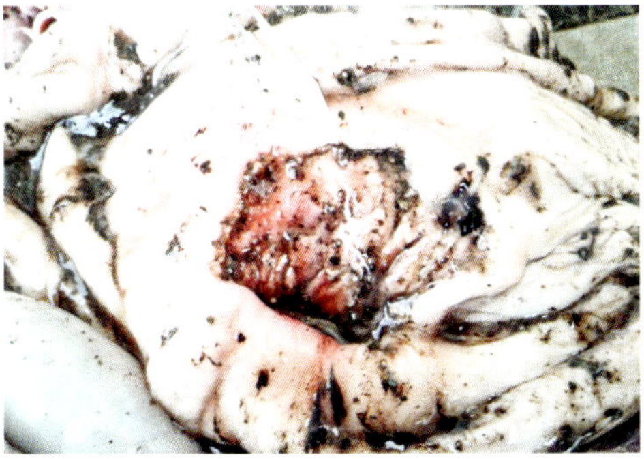

Figure 1 Stomach ulcer in the aglandular area.

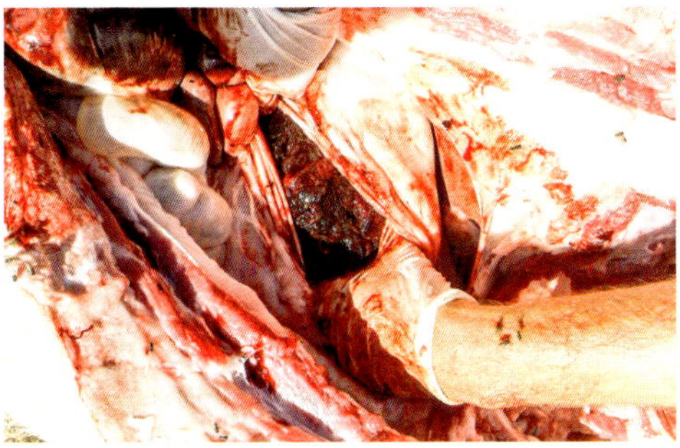

Figure 2 Intragastric haemorrhage caused by ulceration.

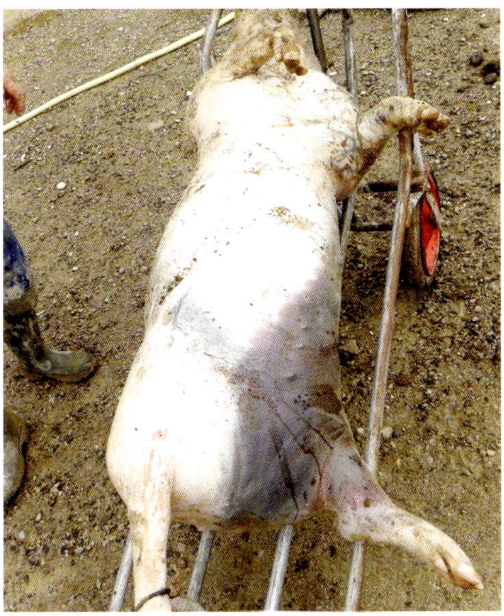

Figure 3 Sudden death in a sow caused by *Clostridium novyi*.

This syndrome is one of the most important causes of mortality in sows. Most deaths occur in the days previous to farrowing and in the first days of lactation, with a larger number of cases in the summer.

The observed lesions are a necrotic liver filled with gas, accumulation of gas in the carcass –the animal's body looks very distended– and fast decomposition (Fig. 3).

The course of the disease is hyperacute and it is therefore difficult to administer a treatment, as the affected sows almost do not show any clinical signs before dying. The whole herd may be vaccinated as a prophylactic measure.

Urogenital infections
Cystitis and pyelonephritis

These diseases are usually the result of ascending bacterial infections. Several bacteria have been isolated from their lesions, such as ***Eubacterium*** (*Corynebacterium*) ***suis*** and ***coliform bacteria***.

The incidence of postpartum urogenital infections, which are often responsible for sudden deaths in sows, is higher in older sows.

To prevent these infections, it is important to achieve a high intake of good quality water and to ensure the sow gets up regularly to urinate. These urogenital infections should not be confused with metritis.

Main diseases of piglets

Gastrointestinal disorders. Diarrhoea

Pigs are monogastric animals with a digestive system quite similar to that of human beings. The food is mixed with acids and enzymes in their stomach in order to be decomposed. Once it has been processed in the stomach, it passes to the intestine, where a process of absorption takes place through the enterocytes, which are part of the villi covering the intestine (Fig. 4).

Diarrhoea is the result of an abnormal functioning of the gastrointestinal system and one of the main causes of mortality in piglets during the lactation period. The affected animals die mainly as a consequence of a hypovolaemic shock due to dehydration. Diarrhoea in piglets is mainly of nutritional or infectious origin.

Nutritional origin

The aetiology of diarrhoea of nutritional origin is very varied. Some authors mention an insufficient colostrum intake as a predisposing factor, as it hinders the development and early maturation of the intestine, in addition to resulting in a deficient immunoglobulin intake.

Conversely, an excessive milk intake may trigger diarrhoea as a result of the animal's incapacity to process the milk completely, since the product passes from the stomach to the intestine too rapidly, before the milk has been efficiently digested in the stomach. This explains why sows with a good milk production and strong piglets are considered to be risk factors of diarrhoea during lactation,

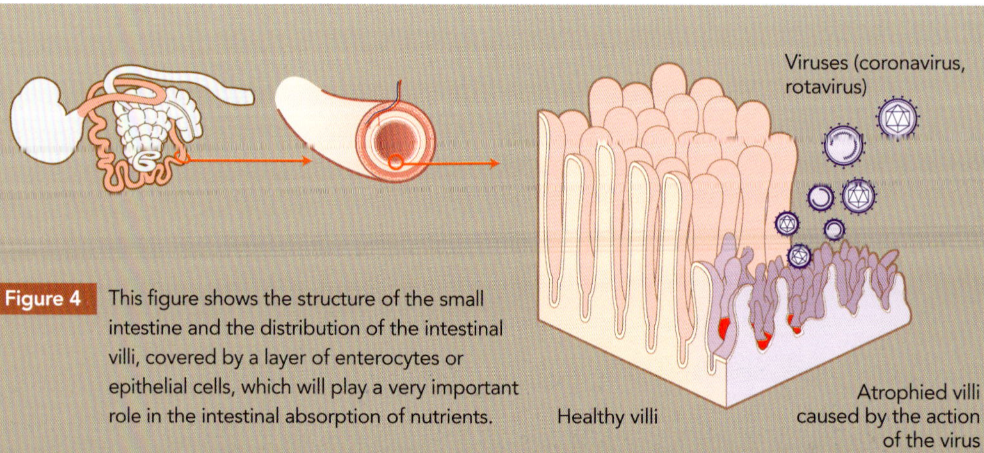

Figure 4 This figure shows the structure of the small intestine and the distribution of the intestinal villi, covered by a layer of enterocytes or epithelial cells, which will play a very important role in the intestinal absorption of nutrients.

as these piglets have a big appetite and access to large quantities of milk. The condition is worsened by the ingestion of milk replacers or prestarters, especially if they are not nutritionally balanced.

Soft faeces may sometimes also be observed instead of diarrhoea. This is due to the consumption of wet food (liquid feeding systems). This is not a pathological problem; it occurs because the large intestine has a limited absorptive capacity. When this capacity is exceeded, the animal cannot absorb more fluids and its faeces have a softer consistency.

An excess of crude protein in the ration can also trigger diarrhoea. It seems to be related to changes in the pH and to a greater predisposition to the proliferation of *Escherichia coli*.

Infectious origin

The most common gastrointestinal disorders of infectious origin causing diarrhoea during lactation are summarised in Table 1.

Table 1 Main infectious agents responsible for diarrhoea in piglets. Adapted from Leman, A.D. *Diseases of the pig*, 1999.

Disease	Agent	Age	Type of diarrhoea	Lesions	IP
Rotaviral infection	Rotavirus	From day 1 until post-weaning period.	Whitish, watery-pasty.	Thinning of the intestinal walls due to moderate atrophy of the intestinal villi.	18-96 h.
Porcine epidemic diarrhoea	Corona-virus	From day 1 until they are adults.	Watery, brownish, and vomiting.	Thinning of the intestinal walls due to severe atrophy of the intestinal villi.	1-8 days.
Transmissible gastroenteritis					1-4 days.
Colibacillosis	*E. coli*	From day 1 until post-weaning period.	Watery, white or yellow.	Intestinal dilatation and congestion of the intestinal walls.	1-3 days.
Clostridial diseases	*Cl. perfringens C*	From day 1 until 14 days of age.	Bloody.	Necrohaemorrhages with gas bubbles.	< 1 day.
Coccidiosis	*Isospora suis*	From day 5 until 15 days of age.	Watery, white or yellow.	Presence of fibrin in the small intestine, enteritis and atrophy of the villi.	4-5 days.

PI: incubation period.

Viruses Bacteria Parasites

Rotaviral enteritis

Rotaviruses are viruses with a tropism for intestinal cells and are part of the enteric pathogens affecting newborn piglets. These ubiquitous viruses are very stable in the environment and resistant to temperature changes, different pH levels, chemical products and many types of disinfectants.

The virus is transmitted by faecal-oral route. The animal ingests the virus, which reaches the small intestine where it invades the enterocytes located at the apex of the villi, thereby damaging or destroying many of them. It results in atrophy of the villi with fusion of some of them (Fig. 4). In general, the degree of atrophy is lower than that caused by TGE virus. The pathogenesis of the disease is very similar to that of the infection by the virus of transmissible gastroenteritis (TGE) and that of porcine epidemic diarrhoea (PED). There is a movement of fluids to the intestinal lumen due to osmosis, which is accompanied by poor absorption and causes diarrhoea. Death is uncommon but it may be related to several factors such as malnutrition, dehydration, an electrolyte imbalance or heart failure.

> There is a relationship between the size of the crypts-height of the villi and the pathogen involved (PED virus, TGE virus or rotavirus).

Susceptible piglets can be infected as a result of viral shedding by carriers, including sows, or because the virus is already present in the environment. They may develop clinical signs or be subclinically infected. Clinical signs appear in the affected animals 12-24 hours after the infection has occurred and include anorexia, apathy, profuse diarrhoea and vomiting. The piglets that overcome diarrhoeic disorders after 3-4 days have a lower growth rate. The clinical signs and lesions are less severe if they are infected at 7 to 21 days of age.

Treatment is symptomatic and involves rehydrating, administering an antimicrobial to prevent any possible bacterial complications and ensuring the animal has access to an area of thermal and environmental comfort. The peritoneal administration of warmed saline solution may sometimes be necessary as a rehydration method. The treatment described can be considered as standard for diarrhoea of infectious origin during the lactation period.

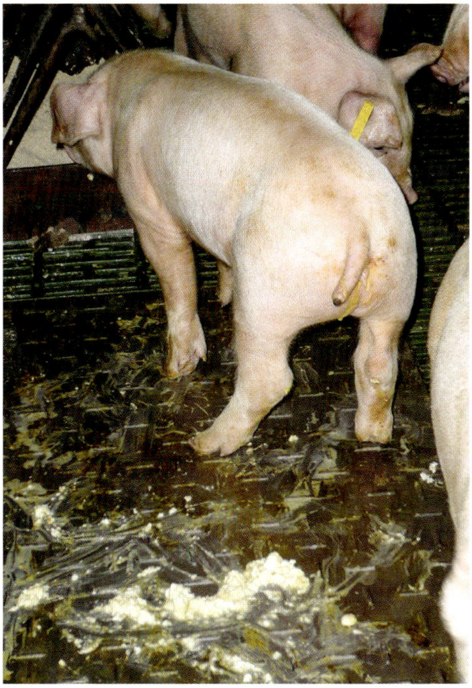

Figure 5 Vomiting and diarrhoea in suckling piglets with PED.

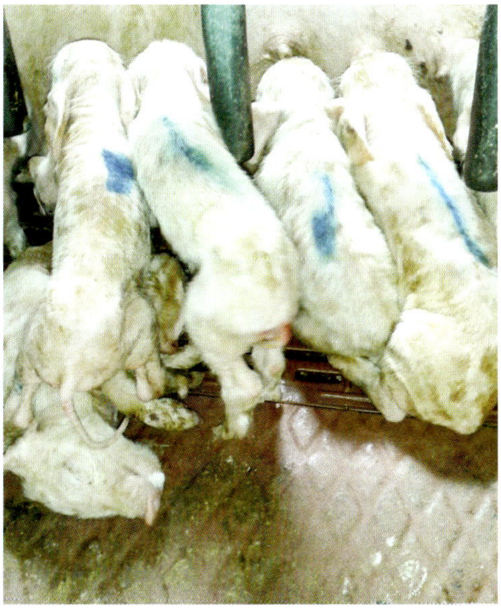

Figure 6 Suckling piglets with diarrhoea caused by the PED virus.

Porcine epidemic diarrhoea (PED)

Caused by a **coronavirus**, its presence worldwide has increased in the past few years due to recent outbreaks of the disease associated with new strains of the virus. It is a highly contagious disease, which has caused very acute outbreaks in some countries such as the USA, with high mortality rates in piglets. As in the case of transmissible gastroenteritis (TGE), PED is caused by a coronavirus, but the two strains have different antigens and there is therefore no cross-immunity between the two diseases. PED is only observed in pigs, it is not a zoonosis and does not affect other animals.

The coronavirus causing PED is very resistant in the environment, which contributes to its spread through livestock vehicles, fomites and materials that have been exposed to contaminated faeces. The main transmission route is thus the faecal-oral route, although the virus has also been detected in semen, blood and nasal content, which may explain why it has a certain capacity to be transmitted by airborne route. The entry of the virus onto farms via porcine plasma (which is included in the composition of milk replacers) seems to have been ruled out, especially if the plasma manufacturing process was correct.

The virus infects the epithelial cells of the small intestine and replicates in them, which causes cell atrophy and degeneration and leads to the shortening of the intestinal villi (Fig. 4). This abnormality hinders the intestinal absorption of nutrients.

Porcine epidemic diarrhoea is highly contagious and has a very acute clinical presentation, similar to that of TGE in naïve herds (epizootic form), with profuse and very watery diarrhoea and vomiting that lead to high mortality rates in piglets of a few days of age (Figs. 5 and 6). The severity of the disease is inversely proportional to the age of the affected animal, since the regenerative capacity of epithelial cells is much lower in piglets of a few hours of life than in older animals. Consequently, the mortality rate during the most acute period of the outbreak in the farrowing unit may vary between 30 and 80 %. Suckling piglets under ten days of age usually die due to the dehydration caused by diarrhoea. The strongest and largest piglets may survive and recover.

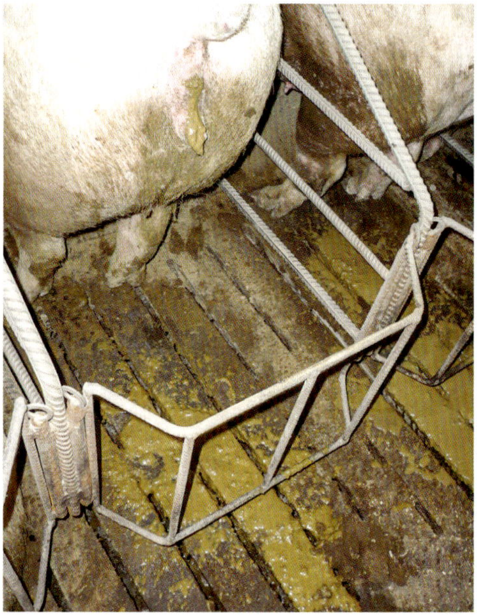

Figure 7 Diarrhoea caused by the PED virus in adult sows.

Sows can also suffer from severe diarrhoea (Fig. 7), with fever and no appetite for several days. This causes the cessation of milk production and the appearance of mastitis, which complicates the viability of the sow's piglets even more. Due to the decrease in the sows' feed intake, their body condition at weaning is poorer and their return to oestrus is delayed for several days.

Diarrhoea in the farrowing unit persists for 2-3 weeks after the acute outbreak, although its intensity is lower. This is due to the formation of subpopulations of naïve animals. Some authors have reported new outbreaks of PED weeks and even months after the initial outbreak. They attributed this to the fact that some sows remained uninfected or to the introduction on the farm of replacement sows that had not previously been infected.

Piglets should receive a symptomatic treatment (identical to that of piglets suffering from diarrhoea caused by rotavirus): rehydration and administration of an antibiotic to avoid any bacterial complications. It is important to provide a source of heat and a dry environment with no draughts. Prevention mainly involves applying good biosecurity measures, since no effective vaccines against this virus are currently available.

Prophylactic measures against coronavirus (PED)

When a veterinary practitioner faces an outbreak on a farm that has not previously been exposed to the virus, all pigs of all ages are susceptible of developing diarrhoea, and the likelihood of a high percentage of suckling piglets dying is high.

Once an outbreak of PED has been confirmed on a farm, a strategy based on the next three key steps should be followed:

1. **Informing.** It is essential to report a laboratory diagnosis of PED virus. This information should be given to the neighbouring farms so they maximise their biosecurity measures. The companies in charge of transporting feed or semen or those dealing with carcass collection should also be informed in order to modify their routes based on biosecurity criteria (the positive farm should be the last stop on the route). The purpose of this first step is to try to keep the disease under control on the farm and to avoid transmission to other operations.
2. **Stabilising the farm**. The purpose is to cause generalised spread of the disease over a relatively short period of time, ten days approximately, to immunise all the animals on the operation. This immunisation should be performed by exposure –or feedback– of the sows to faeces or intestines of viraemic animals (preferably piglets, as they have a higher shedding rate of the virus). It should be ensured that all the sows have had the infection before entering the farrowing unit.
3. **Not introducing replacement sows on the farm.** When an outbreak of PED is diagnosed, it is recommended to postpone the introduction of replacement sows for 4-5 months, so it can be ensured that all the sows have had the infection and none of them are susceptible. If otherwise, this could give rise to subpopulations that may cause new outbreaks.

If these management guidelines are followed, the farm's performance parameters will very likely come back to almost normal levels after three or four weeks, with a significant improvement in the piglets' condition and a considerable reduction in mortality. The possibility of an endemic problem occurring on the farm due to this disease will also be considerably reduced.

Transmissible gastroenteritis (TGE)

Transmissible gastroenteritis (TGE) is a disease caused by a **coronavirus** affecting animals of all ages.

TGE virus is usually transmitted by faecal-oral route, although the airborne route has also been reported as a possible transmission route in animals that are in close contact with each other. The virus is ingested and infects the small intestinal mucosa, thus causing atrophy of the intestinal villi as a result of an important destruction of epithelial cells. This atrophy is responsible for an acute malabsorption syndrome. Severely affected animals eventually die due to dehydration and metabolic acidosis, together with heart failure caused by electrolyte imbalance (in the form of hyperpotassaemia).

Three types of presentation of the disease should be differentiated in function of the immune status of the herd against the coronavirus:

a. **Epizootic disease:** on farms where there has not been any previous exposure to the virus and all the animals are susceptible to be infected, as they have not been immunised. In these cases, the disease causes great losses as it spreads very rapidly and affects all the animals. Piglets suffer from yellowish watery diarrhoea, vomiting, weight loss and dehydration. A high percentage of them die (some authors speak of about 10 % of piglets under a week of age).
   The sows that develop the disease suffer from anorexia and agalactia, which makes it even more difficult for their piglets to survive. Diarrhoea and vomiting may also be observed in some sows.
b. **Enzootic disease:** in herds in which the virus is present and affects replacement animals, which are susceptible of becoming infected when they arrive at the farm. These tend to perpetuate the disease. In this case, piglets also suffer from diarrhoea, although it is less severe, while sows have almost no clinical signs.
c. **Infections in herds that have been previously exposed to the porcine respiratory coronavirus (PRCV)**, a variant of the coronavirus responsible for TGE. When sows are infected with PCRV, their organism develops neutralising antibodies against the coronavirus responsible for gastroenteritis, thereby providing them with immunity. In addition, those animals that have already been infected by PRCV almost do not show any clinical signs and TGE progresses subclinically. In Europe, PRCV has spread very rapidly and widely in swine herds. These have therefore been immunised against the coronavirus responsible for TGE, which does not represent a major problem.

Zinc-deficient diets, immunodeficient animals, low temperatures (the virus resists well to low temperatures, which is why a certain degree of seasonality is observed) are among the main factors predisposing to the disease. Some animals may act as reservoirs, such as dogs, cats and some birds.

There is no treatment against the virus but, as in the case of infections caused by rotavirus and PED coronavirus, the clinical signs may be treated by rehydrating the animals, providing them with a source of heat, ensuring they are dry and administering them an antibiotic against possible complications due to *E. coli.*

Distinguishing an outbreak of PED from an outbreak of TGE is a complex task as they are not very different in terms of their origin, transmission route, mechanism of action, clinical signs, lesions and treatment, although there are some slight differences. The course of TGE is faster due to its shorter period of incubation and more acute presentation, as the intestinal villi are more extensively shortened. Furthermore, the virus causing PED seems to persist more easily on a farm once the acute infection has subsided.

An outbreak of TGE cannot be differentiated clinically from an outbreak of PED, unless laboratory diagnostic techniques are used.

Colibacillosis

Escherichia coli is the most important aetiological agent of neonatal diarrhoea and diarrhoea in suckling piglets. Most of the strains of this bacterium are commensal, that is, they live in the intestine and are not usually harmful to the host, but a reduced number of strains can actually be pathogenic.

The different factors of virulence of *Escherichia coli* have been studied in the past few years. Based on these studies, the different strains have been classified into several pathotypes according to their virulence factors and to pathogenesis of the disease they cause (Table 2).

Table 2 Classification of pathotypes of *E. coli*. Gyles, C.L. and Fairbrother, J.M. *Escherichia coli*. In: *Pathogenesis of bacterial infections in animals* (Ed: C.L. Gyles, J.F. Prescott, J.G. Songer y C.O. Thoen), 4th ed., Wiley-Blackwell, Oxford, UK. (2010).

Pathotype	Disease
Enterotoxigenic *E. coli* (ETEC)	Neonatal diarrhoea, diarrhoea in suckling piglets, post-weaning diarrhoea
Enteroapthogenic *E. coli* (EPEC)	Post-weaning diarrhoea
Shiga toxin-producing *E. coli* (STEC)	Oedema disease
Extraintestinal *E. coli* (ExPEC)	Colisepticaemia, polyserositis, urogenital infections

As can be observed in Table 2, the pathotype responsible for neonatal diarrhoea and diarrhoea in suckling piglets is enterotoxigenic ***E. coli* (ETEC)**. It acts by adhering to the apical surface of the small intestinal epithelial cells in order to subsequently colonise them and produce enterotoxins that modify the flow of water and electrolytes, leading to hypersecretion towards the intestinal lumen. This hypersecretion results in diarrhoea if the animal's large intestine is not able to absorb the excess of fluids. Neonatal diarrhoea and diarrhoea in suckling piglets are therefore hypersecretory. The development and evolution of the diarrhoea depend on several factors, such as:

- **Type of bacteria:** there are many different strains of *E. coli* due to the wide variety of antigens they possess. These antigens determine the pathogenic potential, type of adhesion to the cells and many other characteristics of the bacteria.
- **Host:** the animal's immune status also plays an important role in the development of diarrhoea. The likelihood of the disease appearing in immunodeficient animals is much higher.
- **Environment:** an inappropriate control of the temperature in the farrowing unit causing hypothermia in the piglets may be one of the main triggering factors of the disease. Furthermore, poor hygienic conditions in the farrowing unit also favour the appearance and transmission of neonatal diarrhoea.

The bacteria are transmitted by faecal-oral route. Newborn piglets can be infected only minutes after being born if they come into contact with contaminated faeces of the sow, as they are born with no innate immunity and will not acquire immunity until they have started to ingest their mother's colostrum. In suckling piglets of a few days of age, diarrhoea can develop as a result of a triggering stress factor or combination of these factors affecting the equilibrium between the bacteria and the host.

To be able to transfer immunity against *E. coli* to her piglets, a sow must have generated antibodies against the pathogenic strain present on the operation. Sows should therefore be exposed to these pathogenic bacteria through feed-back during gestation. It is then very important to ensure all piglets drink colostrum so they have minimum antibody levels to fight against these early infections. Diarrhoea is commonly observed in piglets of gilts a few hours after their birth, as these sows have not been sufficiently exposed to the *E. coli* strain present on the farm and cannot transfer immunity to their piglets.

The clinical course of the disease depends greatly on the animal's age:

- **Neonatal diarrhoea:** the affected piglets suffer from severe watery diarrhoea, dehydration, apathy and polyarthritis. The disease results in high mortality rates (Fig. 8).
- **Diarrhoea in suckling piglets:** the animals suffer from moderate diarrhoea and a decrease in their growth rate (fig. 9). The disease has a low mortality rate.

It is essential that sows transfer protective antibodies against *E.coli* to their piglets through colostrum.

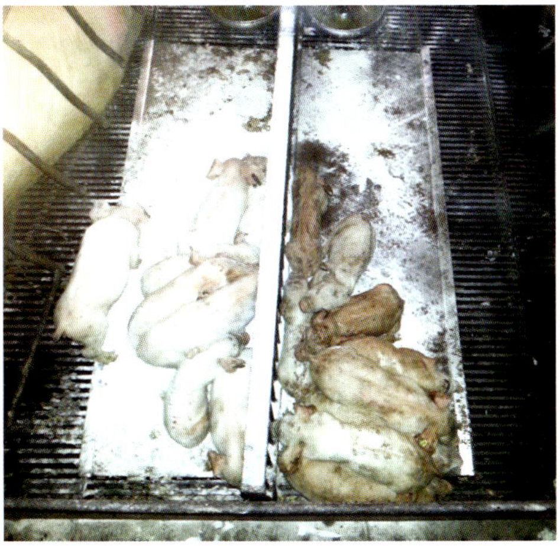

Figure 8 Difference between a litter in which diarrhoea *E. coli* is starting to manifest itself (left) and a litter in which the infection is already established (right).

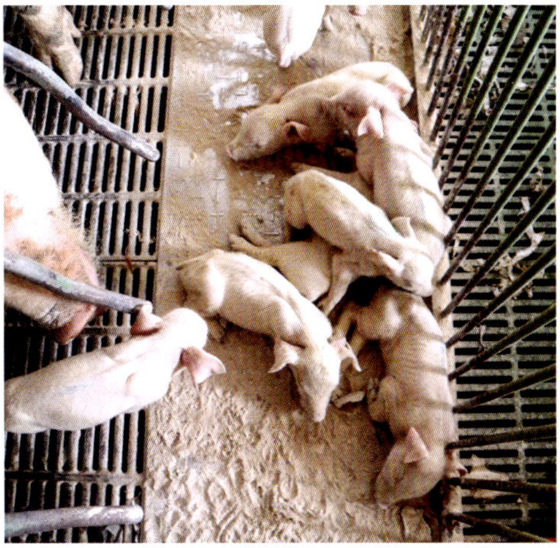

Figure 9 Piglets with delayed growth after overcoming diarrhoea due to colibacillosis.

The necropsy of animals that died without showing any clinical signs of disease reveals dehydration, dilatation of the stomach (which may contain clots of undigested milk) and a small intestine with congestion in its walls.

For a precise diagnosis of the type of *E. coli* present on the farm, rectal samples should be collected using swabs, together with intestinal samples to perform a culture and use the PCR (Polymerase Chain Reaction) method to identify the virulence factors and classify the strain.

The prognosis of the disease is very variable and depends on the age at which diarrhoea appears. Most suckling piglets can recover with appropriate monitoring and care from the farm workers.

Treatment should include an antibiotic chosen based on the results of the antibiogram and rehydration of the animals. It is very important for piglets to have a dry and warm resting area to fight and overcome the infection.

Regarding the prevention of diarrhoea in suckling piglets, it is essential to ensure the sow produces antibodies at the time of farrowing so she can pass them onto her piglets through her colostrum. That is why feedback with infective material is used and vaccines are applied during gestation several weeks before the expected date of farrowing.

When a diarrhoea outbreak occurs on a sow farm, biosecurity measures should be implemented and observed at all times. These measures should include, among others: placing foot baths with a disinfectant at the entrance of each farrowing room, frequently changing needles when litters are processed, not moving piglets with diarrhoea from one litter to another, etc.

Clostridial diseases

C. perfringens

Clostridium perfringens is one of the bacteria responsible for diarrhoea in piglets. There are two main types, type C (CptC) and type A (CptA). This section focuses on *Clostridium perfringens* type C because of its greater pathogenic and damaging potential.

The affected piglets are infected a few hours after being born through the faeces of carrier sows containing pathogenic clostridia. Poor hygiene in the farrowing units increases the likelihood of piglets developing the infection.

When the bacteria reach the small intestine, where they proliferate, they adhere to the enterocytes and produce the necrotising beta-toxin, which causes necrosis and desquamation of the epithelial cells, accompanied by haemorrhage and inflammation. Furthermore, gas is produced and accumulates in the lumen and/or wall of the intestine, thereby causing emphysema.

Clostridium perfringens type C is responsible for an enterotoxaemia characterised by variable morbidity and high mortality rates in newborn and suckling piglets. The clinical signs of *C. perfringens* vary depending on the infective dose, virulence of the bacteria and colostral immunity. The susceptible newborn piglets become sick and may die 4-8 hours after exposure. Piglets infected at more days of age rapidly become weak and are at a great risk of being crushed by the sow; those that survive develop a yellowish-greyish mucoid diarrhoea and have a slower growth rate. In acute outbreaks, piglets may die even before suffering from diarrhoea.

The diagnosis is established at necropsy of the animal. At macroscopic level, a darkening of the skin of the abdominal region and an excess of fluids with blood in the peritoneal cavity and pleura are observed. The lesions usually affect the entire small intestine and parts of the caecum and colon may also be affected, with gas and haemorrhagic fluid in their lumen. Serofibrinous adhesions may be observed between the intestinal loops. In acute cases, the small intestine is necrohaemorrhagic with a deep dark red colour.

Lesions are not as severe if they are caused by *C. perfringens* type A bacteria. Thinning of the intestinal wall is observed and the small intestine is filled with fluid. A culture can be performed as a diagnostic method, while the PCR technique may be used to differentiate CptA from CptC.

Treatment involves the administration of an antibiotic based on the results of the antibiogram. The affected piglets should also be rehydrated and kept in an area of environmental comfort.

As a prophylactic measure, mothers are vaccinated twice during gestation with mixed vaccines against *E. coli* and *Clostridium*, so they can transfer immunity against the toxins to their piglets through their colostrum (the first vaccine is administered halfway through the gestation period and a booster is given 2-3 weeks before farrowing).

Clostridium difficile

Infections by *Clostridium difficile* lead to high mortality rates and have recently grown in significance.

The infection caused by *Clostridium difficile* (Cd) takes place in the piglets' colon and causes diarrhoea with variable morbidity and mortality rates. They usually appear in 1 to 7-day-old piglets. The most pathogenic strains of Cd are known to produce toxins that are associated with the systemic disease causing typhlocolitis and oedema of the mesocolon. The pathogenesis of Cd infections seems to have aspects in common with that of CptA and CptC infections. Cd-related diarrhoea is therefore sometimes difficult to distinguish from that caused by CptA or from neonatal collibacillosis. Laboratory techniques are necessary to diagnose the true aetiology of the process.

The lesions, which occur in the caecum and colon, include oedema of the mesocolon, water content in the colon in addition to, sometimes, respiratory symptoms and/or sudden death.

The treatment for this type of microorganism is the same as that for *Clostridium perfringens*. With regard to its prevention, specific vaccines are available for this strain.

Coccidiosis

Coccidiosis is the term used to refer to the parasitisation caused by several species of protozoa belonging to the genera *Eimeria* (eimeriosis) and *Isospora* (isosporosis). It includes the diseases caused by *Cryptosporidium*, *Sarcocystis* and *Toxoplasma*, although the term coccidiosis is often reserved for the diseases due to *Eimeria* and *Isospora*.

This section focuses on *Isospora suis*, as it is considered as the most important causative agent of coccidiosis during the lactation period.

The parasite has a direct life cycle (there is no intermediate host) and the disease is typical of young piglets, which usually show signs derived from the infestation, although adult animals can also be infected and not shown any signs of it.

The life cycle of *Isospora suis* is detailed in the diagram shown in Figure 10. As can be seen in it, part of the parasite's cycle takes place inside the pig –mainly in the intestinal epithelial cells, where it multiplies and oocysts eventually form through a complex process– while another part of the cycle occurs outside the animal, where the oocysts shed with faeces (up to 400,000 per gram of faeces) acquire their infective capacity as they sporulate.

Oocysts have a great capacity to persist in the environment and can remain viable for up to a year. Under the usual conditions of farrowing units, where the temperature and humidity are high, the sporulation process may take place very rapidly and some sporulated oocysts may already be observed 12-16 hours after their excretion. Most oocysts have sporulated after 48 hours.

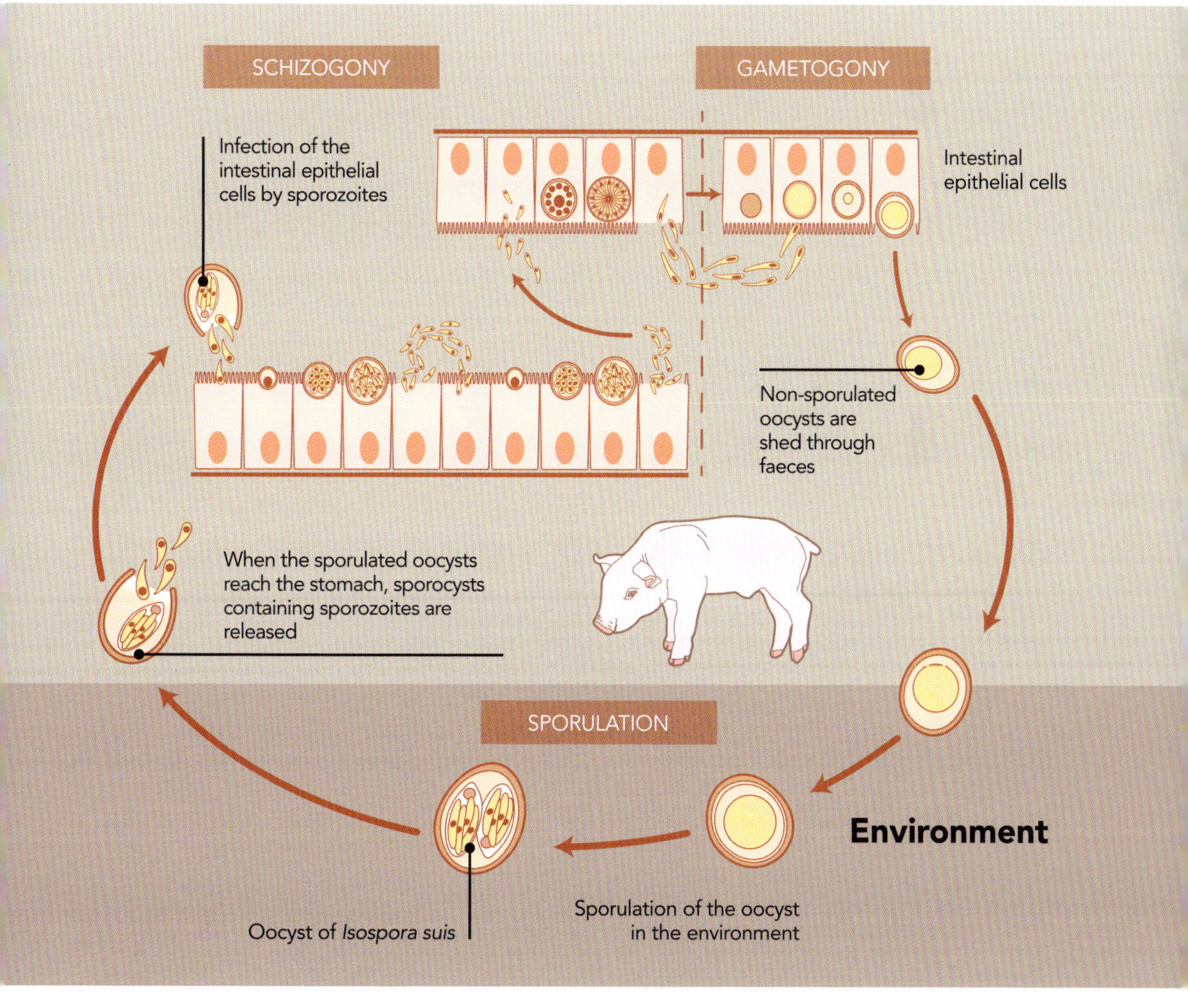

Figure 10 Life cycle of *Isospora suis.*

The animals are infested in the first days after being born. They start to develop a protective immune response from the third week of life, which explains why the incidence of the disease decreases in the post-weaning period. Parasitised piglets are the main source of transmission. In this regard and as has been observed, mothers do not seem to play a decisive role in the transmission of the parasite to their piglets.

It is easy for the parasite to remain on a farm once it is established, as it can be transmitted from one generation of piglets to another if the facilities are contaminated (drinking and feeding troughs, floor...). It has been demonstrated that coccidiosis appears more frequently when farrowing rooms have solid or partially slatted floors instead of fully slatted floors.

The multiplication of the parasite in the animal's intestine causes the destruction of numerous enterocytes due to the different parasitic stages. This prevents the intestinal absorption of nutrients (especially lipids) and water, which leads to diarrhoea, dehydration, loss of electrolytes and a lower growth rate. The affected animals' faeces are of a light yellow colour, foul-smelling and are very characteristic, with a fatty and pasty aspect (Fig. 11) due to the malabsorption of lipids, also known has steatorrhoea or white scours in suckling piglets.

This disease affects animals between 5 and 15 days of age. It is relatively frequent and has a low mortality rate, although it causes growth delays. The degree of pathogenicity depends on the amount of ingested oocysts and on the species involved. This condition usually has a high morbidity rate.

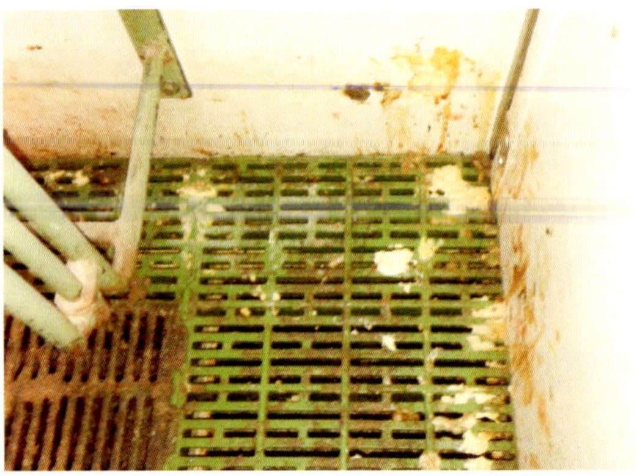

Figure 11 Diarrhoea in piglets caused by *Isospora suis*.

Its diagnosis is simple and inexpensive. It only requires a coprological analysis using a flotation method, which should show sporulated oocysts, and a coproculture to identify the specific species of coccidia.

Prophylaxis is based on the administration of toltrazuril by oral route (20 mg/kg of live weight) at 3-4 days of age, usually at piglet processing.

The administration of a coccidiostatic should be accompanied by proper hygiene measures such as cleaning and disinfection of the farrowing rooms with appropriate products, and by the application of "all-in, all-out" protocols.

Other diseases

Streptococcal infections

Streptococcus suis is a common bacterium in the upper respiratory, reproductive and digestive tracts of pigs. The likelihood of piglets becoming infected is therefore relatively high at farrowing and during the lactation period.

Streptococcal infections usually develop in immunodeficient animals around the time of weaning, but particularly after weaning and rarely before. A study conducted by Reams et al. (1996) described cases of animals affected between 1 and 32 weeks of age, but in 75 % of these cases, the animals were less than 16 weeks old.

The clinical picture shown by affected animals includes fever due to septicaemia, neurological abnormalities such as ataxia and lack of coordination, which usually precede paddling movements, opisthotonus and convulsions associated with meningitis (Fig. 12). *Streptococcus suis* also affects the joints by causing arthritis as well as the respiratory system by causing pneumonia. The typical lesions are fibrinopurulent pericarditis associated with bronchopneumonia and meningitis (Fig. 13).

The diagnosis is established by isolation of the bacteria in combination with the clinical signs and lesions observed in the affected animals, as *Streptococcus suis* is likely to be isolated from the lungs of animals that are apparently healthy. It is easy to confuse streptococcal disease caused by *Streptococcus suis* with Glässer's disease due to *Haemophilus parasuis*, as the clinical picture and lesions shown by affected animals are similar.

Treatment involves the oral or parenteral administration of antibacterial drugs to which the bacterium is sensitive.

Prevention measures should include proper hygiene measures and a good environment in the farrowing pens.

Greasy pig disease (exudative epidermitis)

Staphylococcus hyicus is the pathogenic agent responsible for exudative epidermitis, also sometimes referred to as wet eczema. According to some authors (Martineau, 2011), this bacterium could be related to skin necroses (necrosis of the ears, flanks, tails and facial necrobacillosis as shown in Figure 14).

It affects piglets in the farrowing unit and after weaning. Its incidence is approximately 0.5-1 %. It is associated with states of immunodeficiency such as those due to concomitant diseases, with gilts and with poor environmental conditions – excessive humidity levels reaching more than 60 % and high temperatures with a marked seasonality with more cases appearing in spring and autumn– that facilitate the proliferation of the bacteria. It is also linked to fights between piglets when they are mixed in the farrowing unit, since the resulting wounds can become a route of entry for the bacteria.

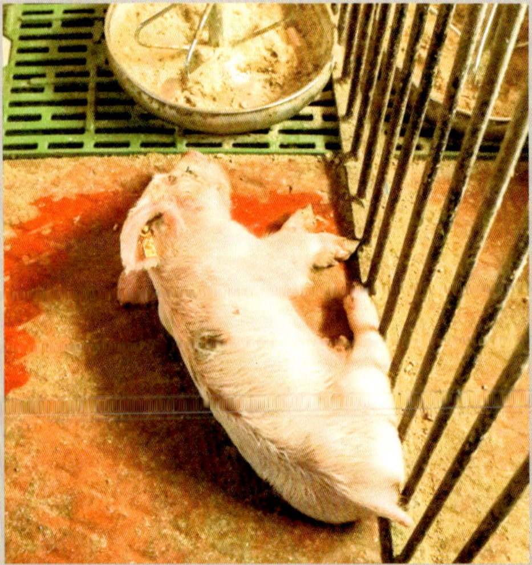

Figure 12 Piglet with clinical signs of meningitis caused by*Streptococcus suis.*

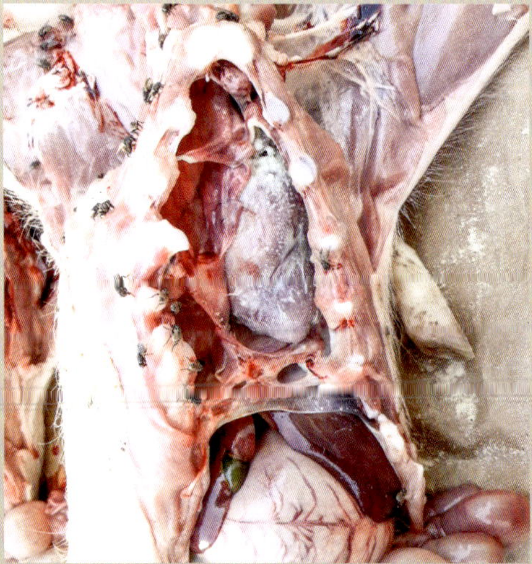

Figure 13 Fibrinous pericarditis and pleuritis compatible with a streptococcal infection caused by*Streptococcus suis.*

There are two main forms of presentation of exudative epidermitis:

- A generalised form, usually in piglets of a few days of age (Fig. 15).
- A multifocal form in older piglets.

The pathogenic action of *Staphylococcus hyicus* lies in the production of exfoliative toxins responsible for the degradation of desmosomes, which are cell structures specialised for cell-to-cell adhesion and thus necessary to maintain the structure of the epithelium.

At the beginning, the skin lesions correspond to focal erosions in the stratum granulosum, which progressively extend to the hair follicles and cause suppurative folliculitis. Sebaceous gland activity increases and produces excess sebum, with the appearance of pruritus, which favours epidermal erosion. Eventually, the excess secretion dries and crusts form with a focal distribution. They tend to coalesce, thereby giving rise to the generalised form. Degeneration and sloughing of the renal epithelium sometimes occurs and results in dehydration. Death is usually observed as a consequence of dehydration and of the loss of proteins and electrolytes.

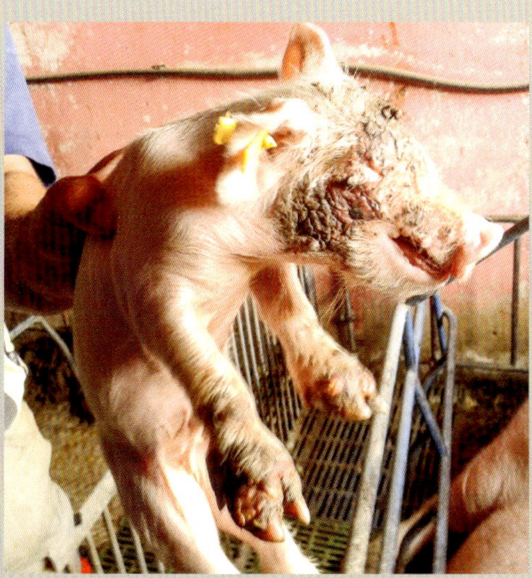

Figure 14 Piglet with facial necrobacillosis caused by *S. hyicus*.

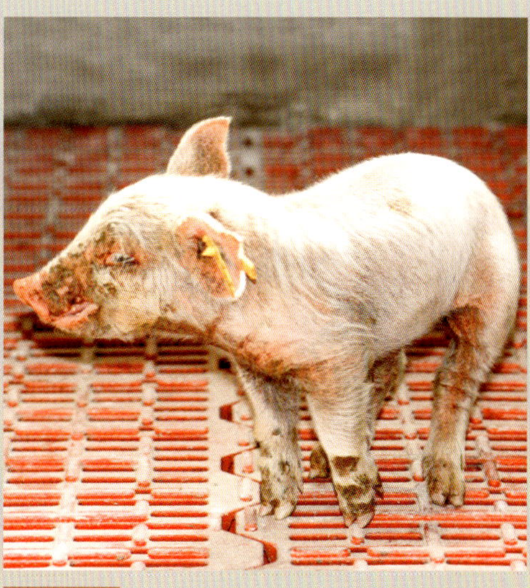

Figure 15 Piglet with lesions typical of exudative epidermitis due to *S. hyicus*.

Animals show apathy, depression and anorexia. Initially, only cutaneous erythema is observed. It is almost imperceptible and usually starts in the axillae and groins, but eventually extends to the rest of the body. Crusts appear after a short time, usually on the head, and tend to coalesce. Ulcers in the mouth and tongue are also observed and the piglets often die after a few days. The disease usually has low morbidity and high mortality rates and can be transmitted from a piglet to its littermates.

> Exudative epidermitis is associated with states of immunodeficiency and with poor environmental conditions (high temperatures and relative humidity levels above 60 %).

Treatment is based on the administration of broad-spectrum antibiotics such as amoxicillin-clavulanic acid or cephalosporins, in addition to chlorhexidine washes and appropriate hygiene and cleaning of the farrowing units and equipment. Systematic teeth clipping is recommended on farms where this disease is widespread.

Joint lesions

It is common to observe suckling piglets with different types of lesions on their limbs and a variable degree of lameness.

Erosions in the area of the carpus are a typical lesion (Figs. 16 and 17). These injuries usually appear on farms with very abrasive floors, when piglets rest their weight on this area in order to suckle. They are more frequent in facilities with iron slatted floors than on operations with plastic slats.

Sometimes, it is also possible to observe lesions and inflammation in the pads or palmar aspect of the hoof, which derive from small erosions that have got infected a few hours after birth.

The crushing of a limb by a mother is another possible cause of lameness. Arthritis and joint lesions are also sometimes observed and caused by infectious agents such as *Streptococcus suis*, *Mycoplasma hyorhinis* and others (Fig. 17).

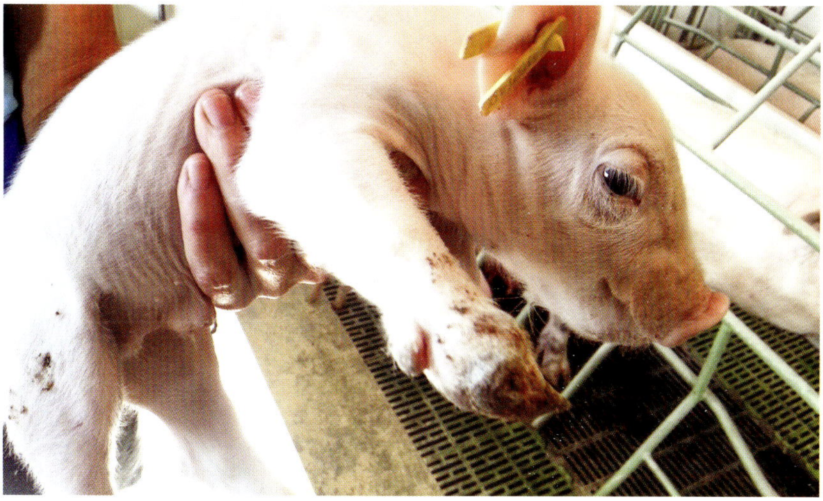

Figure 16 Piglet with a lesion in the area of the carpus, possibly caused by rubbing against abrasive surfaces.

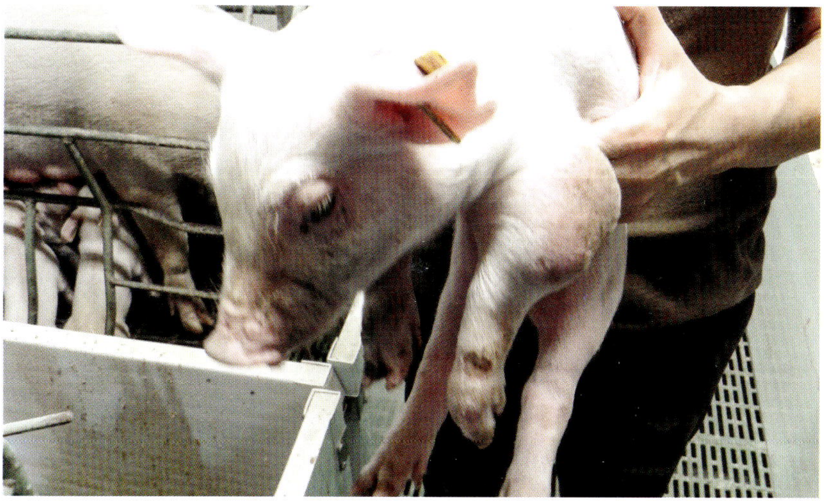

Figure 17 Inflammation of the shoulder joint of infectious origin. A lesion caused by abrasive floors can also be observed on the carpus.

These erosions should be treated with an injectable antibiotic combined with an anti-inflammatory drug, a wound care spray and washes of the affected area with an antiseptic.

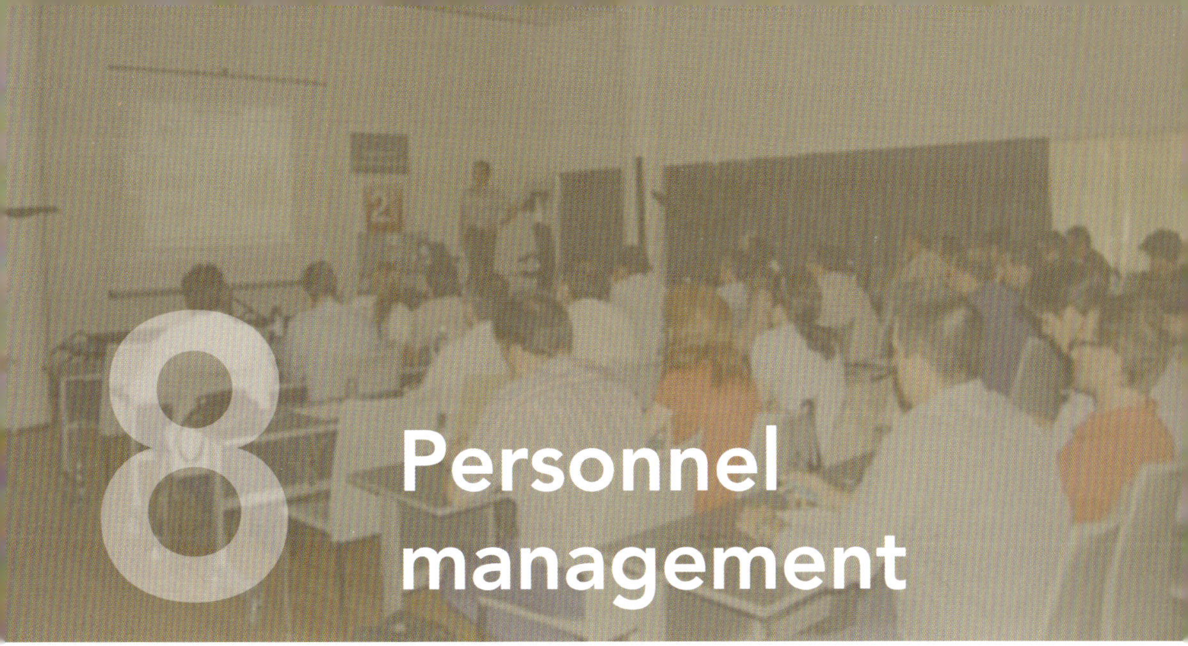

8 Personnel management

The human factor

In an increasingly competitive global market, pig production companies must be highly efficient. One of the elements with a decisive influence on the success of a swine operation is the human factor.

The advances in genetics, nutrition, health and facilities achieved in pig production over the past few years are impressive, but how they are applied to a swine operation remains in the hands of those working on it. It is therefore essential to design a proper personnel management plan, especially at a time when swine operations are increasingly larger and have a greater number of employees.

The three aspects that most determine a pig operation's performance are, in order of importance:

1. Quality of the personnel.
2. Quality of the facilities.
3. Farm's health status.

> The people required to work in farrowing units should be able to ensure lactations take place in an optimal manner after farrowing. The final goal is to wean as many piglets as possible and maximise weaning weight.

With regard to personnel management on a swine operation, it is essential to know and understand a series of essential concepts:

- Selection.
- Training.
- Motivation.
- Skill-building.
- Planning.
- Responsibility.
- Communication.

Figure 1 Importance of the human factor on a swine operation.

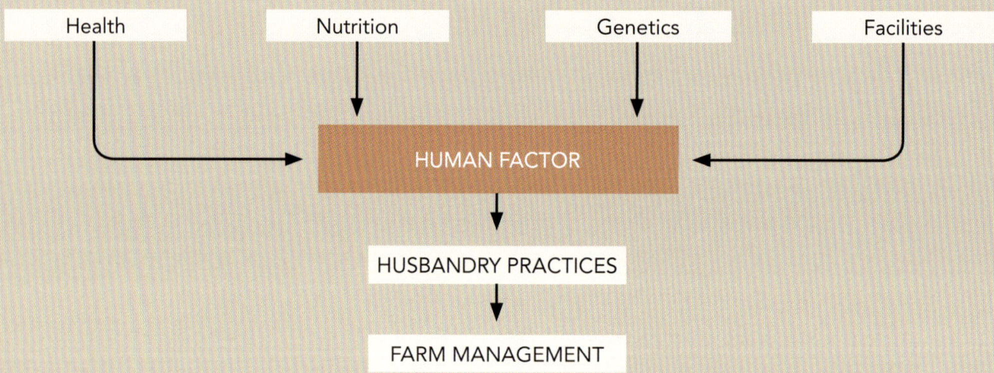

Figure 2 Personnel management in farrowing units: essential concepts.

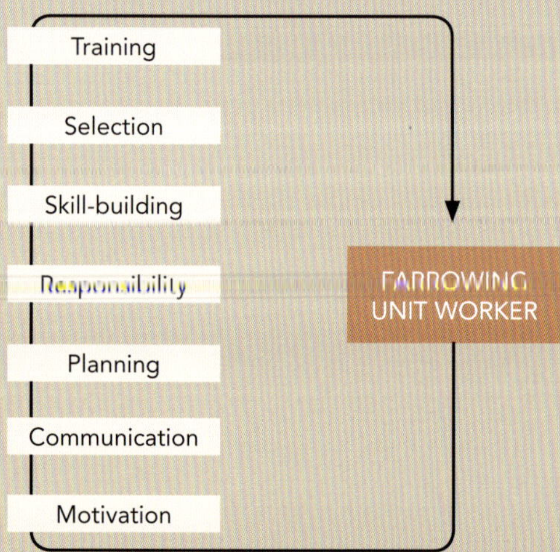

Selection

When dealing with personnel management on a swine operation, the first element to consider is employee selection.

The jobs offered on pig farms entail some disadvantages: rural location, requirement to work every day (including bank holidays and weekends), poor image of the profession, etc. This leads to the first thought of pig farm managers being that "we cannot find anyone".

The key is to offer conditions that are attractive enough for candidates to be interested in the job offered, and with which employee selection can be made based on the farm's needs.

In order to attract young and qualified personnel, it is essential to explain how different the pig industry is from what most people usually tend to think. Farm work is no longer dirty, foul-smelling, too hard work, which does not require any qualifications and is poorly regarded by society. It is an increasingly technical profession that requires training in husbandry and management practices and relies on the use of management software, as farms are more and more automated.

A number of elements need to be clearly defined when selecting personnel:

- Job: tasks to be performed and time to dedicate to them.
- Hierarchical structure of the company and to whom each employee should report.
- Wages and incentives.
- Type of work contract.
- Timetables, weekend shifts, holidays. Flexibility regarding working times, holidays and weekend shifts is vital.

> Appropriate personnel selection does not only lie in finding workers for the operation, but also in correctly assigning each job to a person with the characteristics required to perform it properly.

Training

People are undoubtedly the most important resource in pig production. However, while large amounts of money are often invested in equipment, genetics, nutrition, etc., very little is usually invested in personnel training.

In the current context, with increasingly larger farms where technical knowledge and skills are fundamental and productive performance levels are much higher, both the training and specialisation of the farm personnel are becoming highly relevant, especially of those employees who are going to work in a farrowing unit. The training provided should be divided into a theoretical part and a practical part (Figs. 3 and 4).

A training programme on management practices in the farrowing unit, nutrition, cross-fostering techniques, farrowing assistance, etc. has a very positive short- and medium-term impact on a farm's performance. It is an investment that rapidly leads to improved parameters (Figs. 5 and 6).

Planning a training programme

It is necessary to plan different courses or training levels according to the task each person is going to perform on the operation, or to his/her level of experience or responsibility.

- **Courses aimed at inexperienced workers:** upon completing the training programme, the attendants should perfectly understand the "how" and "why" of all the tasks performed by farm workers.
- **Courses aimed at experienced personnel:** in this case, the training programme should focus on management practices, with a special emphasis on the concepts of farrowing unit management that have a greater impact on the farm's performance.

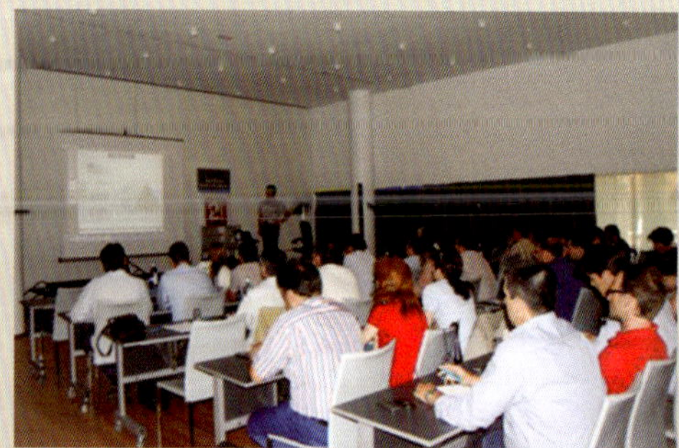

Figure 3 Courses for swine technicians: theoretical training.

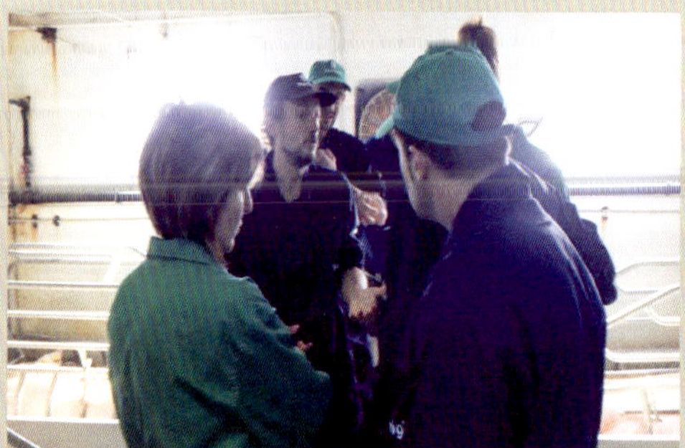

Figure 4 Courses for swine technicians: practical training.

When the courses are given by workers coming from outside the operation, the technical criteria and objectives of the training programme must be clear. This will ensure it is suited to the needs of the swine company for which it has been organised and avoid contradictions between what is said in the course or seminar and the company's guidelines.

Figure 5 Improvement of the parameter "live born piglets" after a training session.

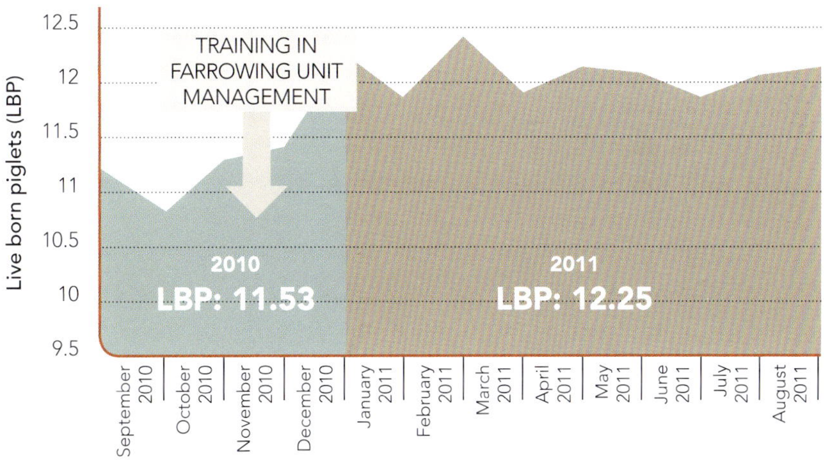

S V CAMPRODON COMA SLP, paper (2012).

Figure 6 Improvement of the parameter "weaned piglets" after a training session.

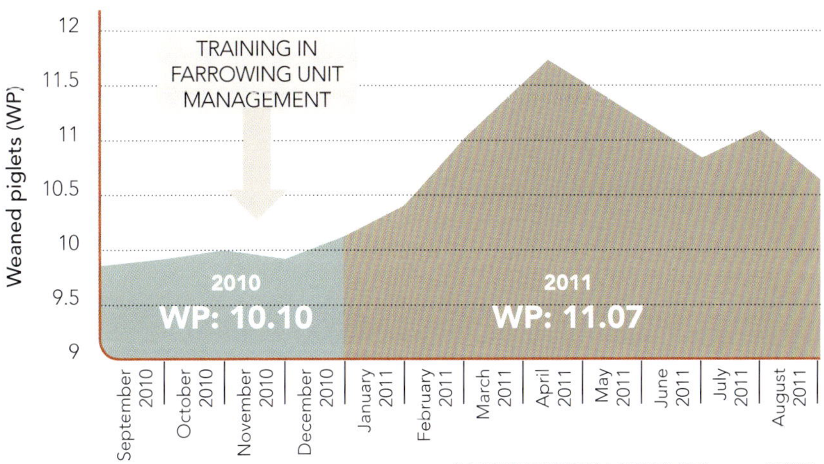

S V CAMPRODON COMA SLP, paper (2012).

Motivation

Motivation is the drive that initiates, directs and maintains behaviour until the desired goal or objective is achieved.

The aim of motivation is to obtain higher performance levels. This is achieved when employees feel comfortable in their job and company; motivation is not always about money, at least not directly. It is necessary for livestock workers to have a more satisfying job in comparison with other industrial jobs, as well opportunities to be promoted.

In our business, it is important to identify the demotivating elements that lead to a job being tedious and unsatisfactory (for example, a poor work environment). At first it is more important to eliminate demotivation than to start a motivational programme for employees.

In order to feel motivated, the personnel need:

- Good salary.
- Good work environment.
- Social benefits.
- Annual holidays and weekend shifts.
- Opportunities to grow as a professional in the company.

Companies satisfy these needs through compensation, which can be of two different types: financial or non-financial.

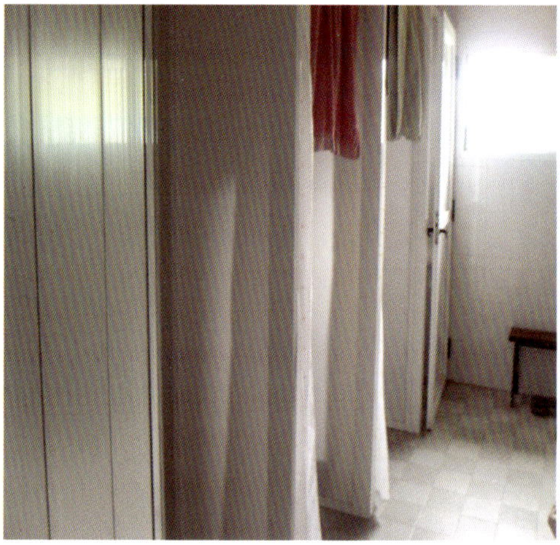

Figure 7 Changing rooms in good condition, favouring a good work environment.

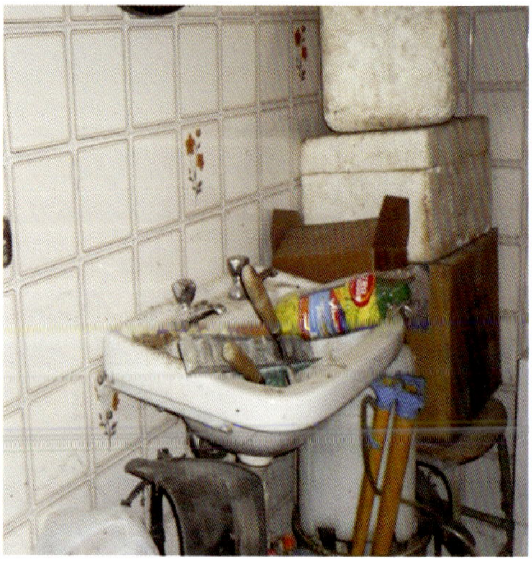

Figure 8 Changing room in very poor condition, favouring a poor work environment.

Financial compensation

Financial compensation is that which provides employees with economic benefits, either directly (wages and incentives) or indirectly (insurances, health services, paid holidays, etc.).

Non-financial compensation

Non-financial compensation provides the employee with another series of benefits that are also very important when it comes to maintaining high levels of motivation: personal satisfaction when the job is well done, decent working conditions, with a changing room, eating area and work clothes in good condition, etc. (Fig. 9).

Figure 9 Types of compensation. From Collell, M. Motivación y organización del trabajo, *Suis*, 2006.

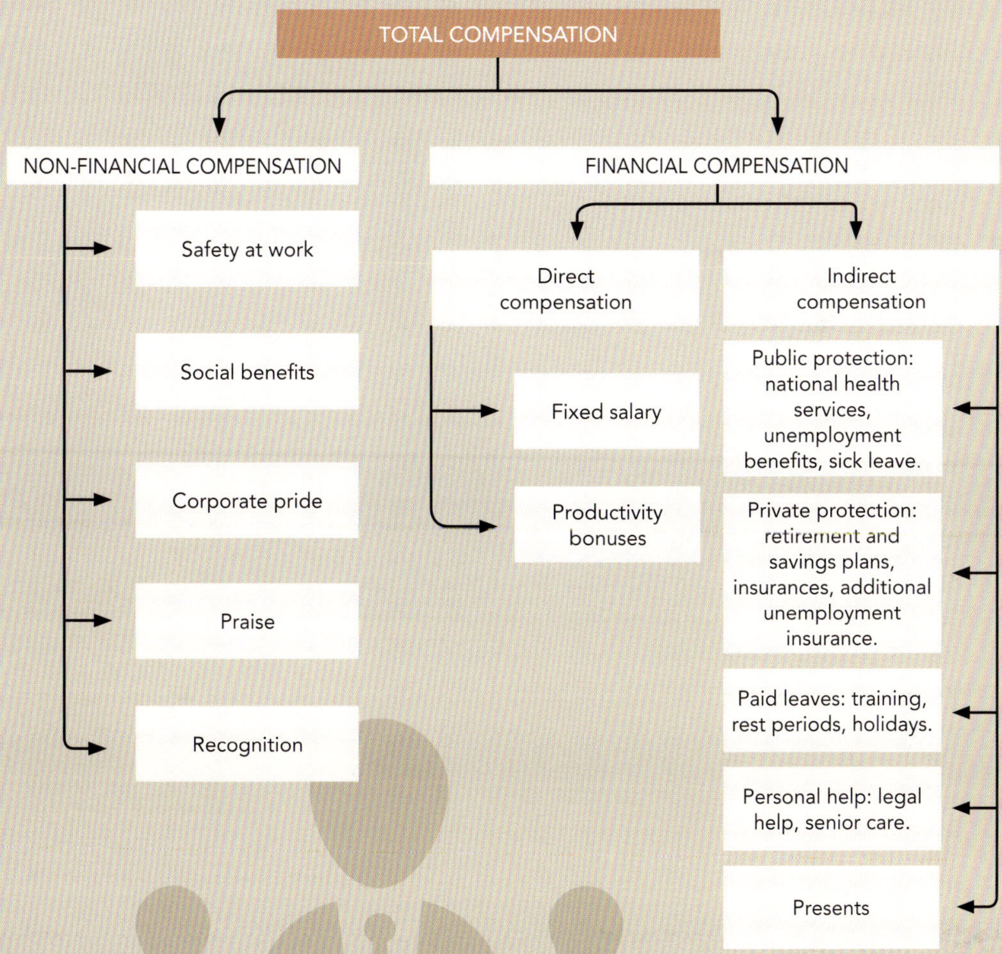

Skill-building

Skill-building is the acquisition of technical knowledge, both theoretical and practical, to allow employees to perform specific tasks or activities with greater efficiency, in this case in all the areas associated with lactation in the sow.

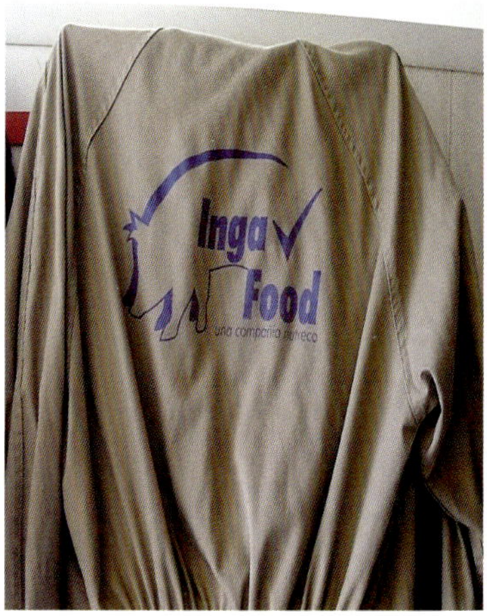

Figure 10 Work clothes with the company's name, which promotes identification with a project.

Tasks associated with lactation

1. Piglet processing: several actions have to be carried out, such as iron injections, tail docking, possible antibiotic treatments, early vaccinations.
2. Cross-fostering: evening out litters and leaving every sow with an appropriate number of piglets according to her history, ensuring fostering of runt piglets, etc., and placing any extra piglets with nurse sows.
3. Sow feeding management: feeding, cleaning the troughs of the sows that have not finished their ration, adjusting the dispensers individually to increase, maintain or decrease the ration, adding water (Fig. 11b).
4. Piglet feeding management: ensuring they drink enough colostrum and nurse correctly, placing pans for creep feed and providing small amounts of feed (creep feeding).
5. Daily health monitoring of sows: possible mastitis or agalactia, anorexia, lameness, injuries, fever. Antibiotic and/or analgesic and/or antipyretic treatment for each case.
6. Daily health monitoring of piglets: piglets with diarrhoea, lameness and corresponding treatment (antibiotics, rehydration, anti-inflammatory drugs, etc.), deaths.
7. Daily cleaning and sweeping of the aisles in the farrowing unit to maintain good overall hygiene.
8. Daily cleaning of the rear part of the stalls to remove faecal material (Fig. 11a).
9. Systematic vaccination of sows and piglets during lactation (for instance, vaccines against parvovirus and erysipelas in sows and against circovirus in piglets, Fig. 11c).
10. Daily recording of the tasks performed, as well as of the sows with problems, cross-fostering procedures, etc., and data collection and recording using a farm management software.

The need for skill-building arises when there are differences between what someone should know to carry out a task and what he/she actually knows.

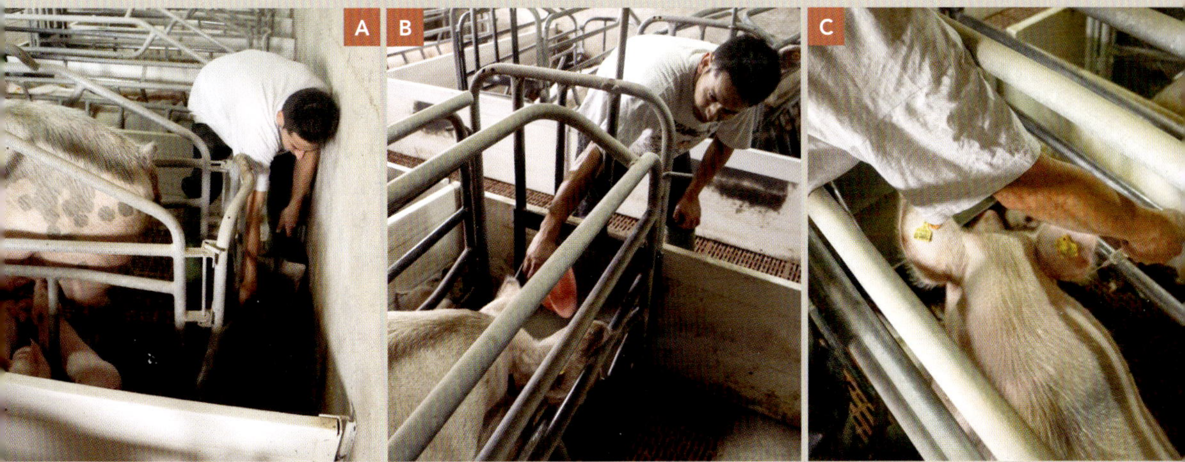

Figure 11 Tasks associated with lactation: cleaning the rear part of the stalls (a), cleaning the feeding troughs (b), vaccinating mothers (c).

The learning process of new workers on a farm includes several steps:

- **Managing:** new employees are shown their specific tasks on the operation.
- **Supervising:** they perform these tasks under supervision.
- **Showing trust:** once they perform their tasks satisfactorily, they should feel trusted to carry them out.
- **Delegating:** new workers reach the skills required to perform the tasks and make decisions relating to their daily work. They are directly responsible for their work and a supervisor monitors their results.

The main tools to achieve skill-building are training and experience.

Planning

Work should be planned on farms in a way that allows all workers to know clearly what tasks they have to perform as well as when, how and how long they should take to carry them out.

> A work schedule is a tool that allows the systematic organisation of relevant information to correctly perform a task.

As a planning tool, a work schedule will allow farm managers to define job descriptions, choose supervisors and set goals and global objectives.

Responsibility

Responsibility is a concept related to people's capacity to accept the consequences of their acts.

Anyone who makes a decision should also face its consequences and be responsible for the tasks performed.

Workers in a farrowing unit should accept the responsibility for the results of the tasks they are asked to perform and for whether the set objectives are achieved.

Communication

On pig farms, particularly on larger, industrial-type operations with a larger number of workers, communication policies are increasingly important. This will contribute to keeping the personnel working on the farm motivated and focused on their job.

Three types of communication have been defined according to the direction in which messages are transmitted: downward, upward and horizontal communication.

> Communication should never be unidirectional, as two of the most important benefits of the process would be lost: response and interaction.

Downward communication

The information comes from the farm managers and goes down to the different levels of the hierarchy. A variety of communication tools are available: employee handbook, handbook of good practices, informative meetings, interviews, group emails, etc.

Upward communication

These are the messages that are transmitted from the lower levels of the hierarchy to the upper levels, and which allow employees to raise issues and make suggestions. This type of communication can be encouraged by means of regular meetings, suggestion boxes, email, etc.

Horizontal communication

It occurs between people at the same level in the operation's hierarchy. It is usually a more informal type of communication and promotes collaboration and teamwork.

Personnel turnover

An important concept to bear in mind on swine operations is the personnel turnover rate, which is sometimes high. In order to calculate the personnel turnover rate (PTR), it is only necessary to know the average number of people who have worked on the operation over the past year and the number of people who have either resigned or been made redundant, without taking into account those who have retired, are on sick leave, or deceased employees.

$$\text{PTR} = \frac{\text{Number of separations (resignations or redundancies)}}{\text{Average number of employee during the year}} \times 100$$

The personnel turnover rate (PTR) indicates the degree of satisfaction of employees with their job on the operation. It is highly variable and depends on many factors (salary, work environment, etc.). Some experiences point out that companies with good remuneration policies are those that obtain better results and where personnel turnover is lowest.

Teamwork

On increasingly larger operations with a greater number of employees, the concept of teamwork becomes highly relevant.

The performance results of each area on the operation (services, farrowings, lactation) depend on how well tasks are performed in the other areas (for example, prolificacy depends on successful insemination of the sows, successful insemination depends on their body condition at weaning, etc.). It is important for swine farm workers to clearly know they are all part of a team and that their work affects that of the others, and therefore the overall productivity of the operation.

> In order for a team to work effectively, there must be a leader. The leader is the person who gives shape to the structure of each group. In the case of a sow farm, the leader should ideally be the farm owner or manager.

A farm manager's objective is to optimise profits. With a global view, he/she should form groups of people who work well as a team and each have individual responsibilities, but who all look and work towards a common goal: achieving maximum productive performance levels on the farm.

The difference between a group of people and a work team determines the efficiency of a company.

Working with objectives

A way of motivating the farm personnel and controlling production is to work with measurable weekly or monthly production objectives for each area of the farm (farrowings, gestation, services). They may be either individual or group objectives for the whole team.

In order to establish objectives, it is necessary to follow **S.M.A.R.T.** criteria:

- **S**pecific.
- **M**easurable.
- **A**chievable.
- **R**ealistic.
- **T**ime-based.

SMART objectives will be defined based on the farm's real productive levels and on those the farm manager wants to reach. In the case of farrowing units, these objectives should essentially be based on these parameters:

1. Live born piglets.
2. Stillborn piglets.
3. Birth-to-weaning mortality rate.
4. Weight of weaned piglets.

Among these parameters, the weight of weaned piglets per farrowing and birth-to-weaning mortality rate are those that best assess the quality of the work carried out during the lactation period. These objectives encourage and motivate employees, not only for financial reasons, but also because they will take pride in a job well done.

An incentive pay scheme should be designed together with the objectives, based on a fixed pay with a variable bonus that will increase depending on whether good results are obtained with regard to these parameters. The farm manager should also set payment brackets (productivity bonuses) corresponding to specific data related to the parameters that are evaluated.

> A good incentive pay scheme for workers in a farrowing unit will improve the farm's technical and economic performance.

Table 1 Example of an incentive pay scheme for workers in a farrowing unit.

Birth-to-weaning mortality rate (%)	Monthly bonus	Weaned piglets/litter	Monthly bonus	Kg weaned/ litter	Monthly bonus
9-10	–	≤ 10	–	60-65	–
7-8	50 euros	10 to 11	50 euros	65-70	50 euros
5-6	100 euros	11 to 12	100 euros	70-75	100 euros
≤ 5	150 euros	≤ 12	150 euros	75-80	150 euros

Thus, a worker in a lactation unit can earn up to 450 euros per month in incentives if he/she achieves a mortality rate < 5 %, weans more than 12 piglets per farrowing and reaches between 75 and 80 kg of weaned piglets per litter.

Occupational health and safety

Many countries have labour laws that oblige business managers to inform their workers about the health hazards associated with their profession, as well as about the preventive measures they should implement to avoid them.

For a business manager, the most effective way of covering this need is to carry out occupational risk assessments, which may be mandatory depending on their national legislation.

A list can be made of the general and specific risks that need to be addressed through a series of preventive measures (Table 2).

Both general and specific preventive measures should be adopted regarding these risks.

Table 2 Main occupational risks in farrowing units.

General risks	Specific risks
Lack of order and hygiene in work areas.	Farm facilities in poor condition.
Exposure to external environmental conditions. Heat and cold.	Risks associated with handling animals.
Heavy lifting (feed sacks, etc.).	Working alone.
Road safety on the way to the operation and back.	Risks associated with the use of veterinary instruments.
Loud noises.	Risks associated with the use of chemical products.
	Risks associated with biological agents.

Rules to prevent work accidents

The ten golden rules for risk prevention at work are listed next.

- Before starting:
  1. Get informed about the tasks that need to be performed.
  2. Think about the risks that may exist.
  3. Ask for the necessary tools and protective equipment.

- While working:
  4. Respect health and safety signs.
  5. Use personal protective equipment.
  6. Take care and respect collective protection equipment.
  7. Do not run unnecessary risks.

- At the end of the working day:
  8. Leave tools and protective equipment ready for use.
  9. Think: “Have we worked safely?”.
  10. Remember: “Safety begins with oneself!”.

Personal protective equipment

The farm owner must provide all the employees with the necessary personal protective equipment, such as safety boots, masks, gloves, hearing protectors, etc.
In addition, clear directions should be given on what to do in case of emergencies, such as fires, accidents requiring first aid, etc.

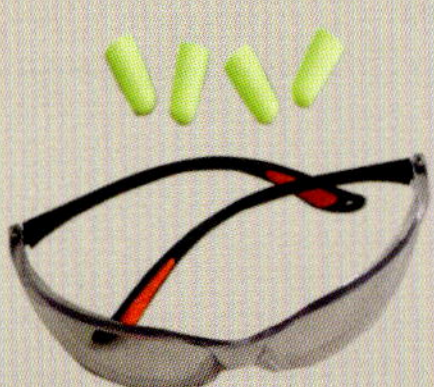

Hearing protectors and safety goggles

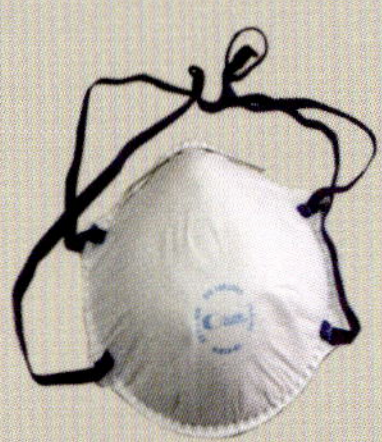

Particulate respirator

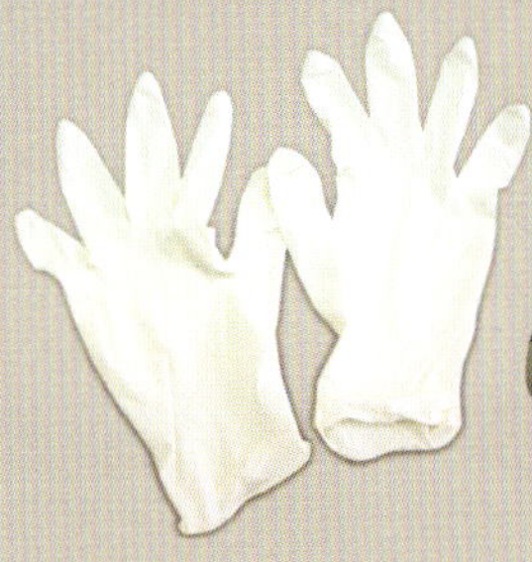

Latex gloves

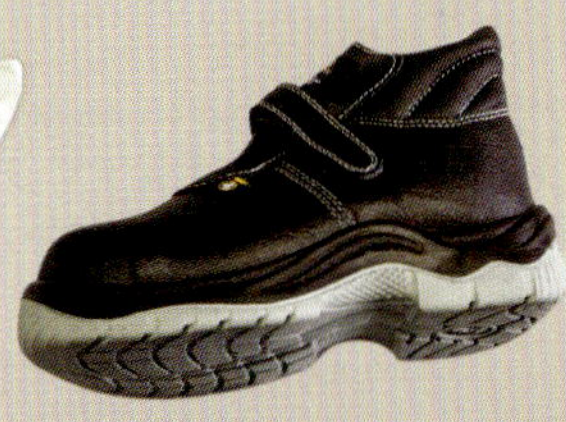

Safety shoes with protective reinforcement in the toe

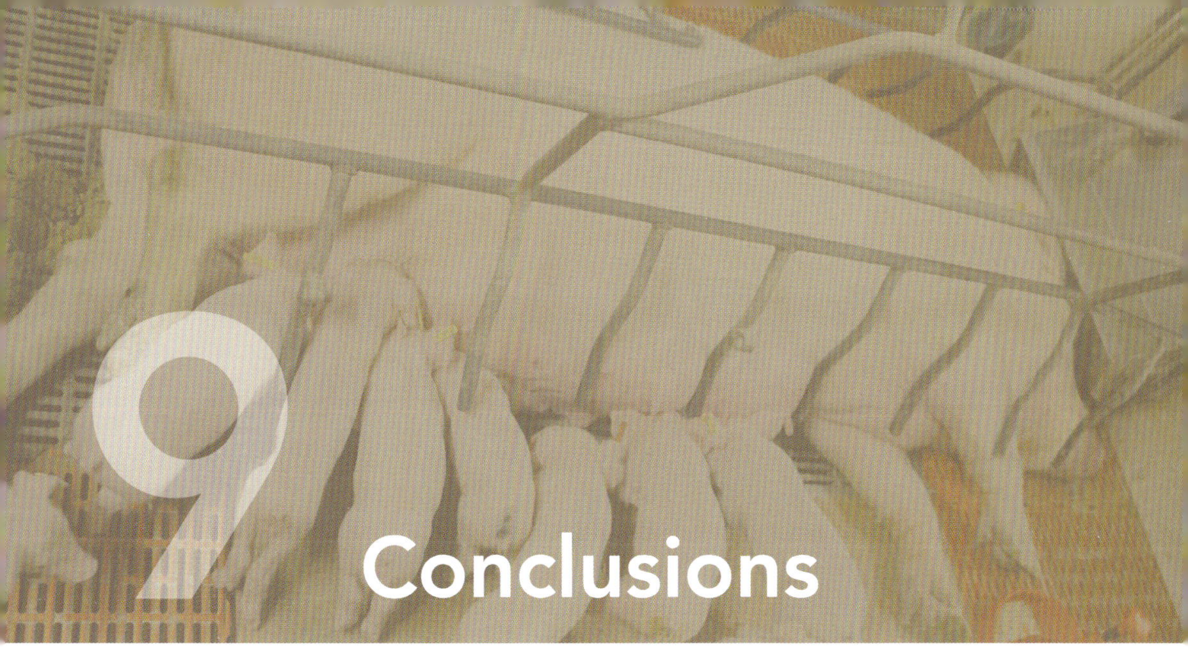

9 Conclusions

As a summary of all the topics addressed in this book, the following conclusions should be highlighted:

- The new hyperprolific lines of sows are capable of farrowing large litters, but these are much more heterogeneous and piglet weight at birth is lower. Moreover, the number of functional teats and milk production of these sows are insufficient for them to nurse all the live piglets they farrow. To solve this new situation, two types of strategies are mainly applied:
  - **Some based on providing more natural milk to piglets**.
  - **Others based on providing supplementary feed to piglets**.

  In most cases, a combination of both strategies is used.
- The purpose of nutrition during the lactation period is to maximise litter weight at weaning, which depends on the number of weaned piglets and their weight. To achieve this objective, which some genetics companies set at 200 kg of weaned piglet per sow and year, sows must produce as much milk as possible. Modern sows are much leaner than 15-20 years ago; they also have a higher body weight in relation to their age and keep growing throughout the lactation period, which results in greater maintenance requirements.
- New nutrition strategies try to minimise the loss of body condition during lactation by favouring feed intake in this phase. Once farrowing is finished, sows should reach a high feed intake as soon as possible to avoid a loss of body condition and favour milk production.
- A sow should not lose more than 10 % of her body weight during lactation and her backfat thickness should not be reduced by more than 3 mm. Greater losses compromise the following reproductive cycles by prolonging

the weaning-to-service interval and worsening future fertility and prolificacy. Sows should be fed two to three times a day.

- To maximise sow feed intake, it is essential that sows drink a lot of a water, up to a maximum of 40-50 litres daily. For this reason, drinking water systems should provide a flow rate of 4-6 l/min minimum.
- Feeding curves for lactating sows should be designed by monitoring their feed intake and adjusted to their body condition, genetics and age, as well as to the number of piglets in their litter.
- Sow feeding at any productive phase –especially during lactation– should be controlled individually taking into account the sow's body condition, which should be monitored regularly, and her physiological stage.
- Feeding protocols should be clear and simple. They should be known and understood by all the farm workers, as these are responsible for adjusting feed dispensers taking into consideration the density variations of feed.
- The main food for piglets during lactation is their mother's milk. However, it does not provide all the nutrients they need to express their maximum genetic growth potential. That is why, from 10-14 days of age, piglets are administered solid supplementary feed, which promotes the development of their digestive tract and contributes to a reduction in the atrophy of their intestinal villi at weaning.
- It is cheaper to produce kilograms of piglet when piglets are fed by their mother to achieve a higher weaning weight, than when they are given feed and other nutritional supplements.
- The environment in farrowing units should be quiet to favour a good farrowing process and lactation. For this to be possible, it is essential to strictly comply with environmental and comfort conditions for sows and piglets.
- Productive performance can be improved with better knowledge of the environmental needs of sows and piglets and automated environmental control systems in the farrowing unit.
- Colostrum intake is fundamental. All piglets must drink colostrum from their mother in a sufficient amount in their first hours of life. To facilitate this process, techniques such as alternate nursing are applied.
- It is recommended to process piglets on their third day of life, when they are more viable and cope better with stress.
- Castration is carried out on many farms in order to eliminate boar taint in carcasses and obtain higher-quality meat products.
- The best time to castrate piglets is at approximately 4-6 days old. The European legislation on animal welfare is very strict and prohibits the castration of piglets over 7 days of age without anaesthesia.

- In the future, less invasive methods for castration will be applied, such as immunocastration.
- Cross-fostering is the method that best adapts to operations with hyperprolific sows, as they optimise farm productivity by taking advantage of the available resources.
- The choice of a fostering system on a farm depends on prolificacy, and, to a lower extent, on the facilities (number and type of farrowing places) and the personnel's technical abilities and qualification.
- The isowean (isolated weaning) principle, which involves producing piglets using early, medicated and segregated weaning, revolutionised pig production worldwide and favoured early weaning under 21 days of age to prevent the transmission of many diseases from sows to their piglets. These theories are partly outdated and weaning today is usually done between the 3rd and 4th week of life.
- On operations with health control programmes, weaning at 28 days of age is the most recommended option as a higher weaning weight is achieved, so that piglets start to eat earlier and have a faster growth rate as well as fewer digestive disorders.
- Piglets weaned at about 21 days of age weigh between 6 and 6.5 kg, while those weaned at 28 days of age weigh between 8 and 9 kg, which facilitates subsequent management practices such as wean-to-finish management.
- According to the current European legislation on animal welfare, piglets should not be weaned at less than 28 days of age, unless a veterinary practitioner recommends they are weaned earlier as an exceptional measure for the control and/or eradication of a disease, and provided they are taken to facilities specially prepared for this purpose.
- The objective in terms of health in lactation is to produce piglets with the highest health status possible. This will have an impact on the number of weaned piglets per farrowing, their quality and their subsequent growth in the fattening period.
- A good preventive policy improves the health status of the operation, resulting in healthier piglets and a better technical and economic performance.
- A health strategy should be defined for each operation depending on its health objectives, with a set of measures that should include biosecurity and parasite control measures as well as vaccination plans and systematic treatments.
- The advances achieved in swine genetics, nutrition, health and facilities in the past few years are spectacular, but how they are applied depends on

the farm personnel. Farrowing unit workers must be able to ensure that, after farrowing, the lactation period takes place in an optimal manner in order to wean as many piglets as possible with an appropriate weaning weight.

- The concept of teamwork is highly relevant on swine operations, which are increasingly larger and haver a greater number of employees.
- Appropriate personnel selection does not only lie in finding workers for the operation, but also in correctly assigning each job to a person with the characteristics required to perform it properly.
- Training and specialisation of the farm personnel is key, especially of those who are going to work in farrowing units. Training programmes should include a theoretical part and a practical part on new husbandry practices in farrowing units.

Bibliographical references

DEPARTMENT OF AGRICULTURE, FORESTRY AND FISHERIES, REPUBLIC OF SOUTH AFRICA. Management. Piglets from birth to weaning [online]. Department of Agriculture, Forestry and Fisheries, Republic of South Africa, 2014 [accessed 2014]. Available from: http://www.nda.agric.za/docs/Infopacks/management.htm

AHERNE, F. Feeding the lactating sow [online]. The Pig Site, November 2001 [accessed 2014]. Available from: http://www.thepigsite.com/articles/493/feeding-the-lactating-sow

AKEY COMPANY. Split-suckling: a technique designed to reduce preweaning mortality. *Swine newsletters*, Brookville, 2003.

ASSOCIATION OF SWINE VETERINARY PRACTITIONERS OF ARAGON. *Manual de prevención de riesgos laborales*, 2006.

BARCELO, J., PAZ, X. *Fallo lactacional de la cerda.* Barcelona: Merial, 2005.

BELENGUER, P. et al. *Chequeos y árboles de decisiones en reproductoras y lechones*. Barcelona: Temis Medical, 2014.

BOVEY, K.E. et al. The effect of birth weight and age at tail docking and ear notching on the behavioral and physiological responses of piglets. *Journal of Animal Science*, 2014, 92 (4): 1718-1727.

BUFFONY, L. et al. Coccidiosis neonatal de los lechones. *Albéitar,* 2014, 180: 6-8.

BUTLER, J.E. Immunologic aspects of breast feeding, antiinfectious activity of breast milk. In: T. K. Oliver and T. H. Kirschbaum (eds). Human Lactation. *Semin. Perinatol.* 3:255.

BUXADE, C. et al. *La cerda reproductora: claves de su optimización productiva*. Madrid: Mundi-Prensa, 2008.

BUXADE, C. AND LÓPEZ, D. *Bienestar animal y ganado porcino: mitos y realidades.* Madrid: Mundi-Prensa, 2005.

BUXADE, C. et al. *Producción porcina: aspectos clave.* Madrid: Mundi-Prensa, 1999.

CARRERA, R. et al. Influence of birth order, birth weight, colostrums and serum immunoglobulin G on neonatal piglet survival. *Journal of Animal Science and Biotechnology*, 2012: 3-42.

CALLEJO, A. AND OVEJERO, I. *Control ambiental de instalaciones de ganado porcino*. Barcelona: Merial, 2007.

CAMPRODON, A. AND COMA. E. *Cerda hiperprolífica. Manejos generales.* Technical meeting Inga Food-S. V. Camprodon SLP, Ceva, Zaragoza, Spain, 2012.

CASANOVAS, C. Cerdas nodrizas (I) [online]. 3tres3, December 2012 [accessed 2014]. Available from: http://www.3tres3.com/consejos_de_manejo/cerdas-nodrizas-i_31845/

CASANOVAS, C. Cerdas nodrizas (II) [online]. 3tres3, February 2012 [accessed 2014]. Available from: http://www.3tres3.com/consejos_de_manejo/cerdas-nodrizas-ii_32002/

CASANOVAS, C. Cerdas nodrizas (II) [online]. Mover cerdas "hacia atrás" [online]. 3tres3, June 2013 [accessed 2014]. Available from: http://www.3tres3.com/consejos_de_manejo/cerdas-nodrizas-iii-mover-cerdas-"hacia-atras"_32408/

CASANOVAS, C. Traspasos de lechones hasta 3-4 días post parto [online]. 3tres3, October 2012 [accessed 2014]. Available from: http://www.3tres3.com/consejos_de_manejo/traspasos-de-lechones-hasta-3-4-dias-post-parto_31469/

CASANOVAS, C. Traspasos de lechones hasta 3-4 días post parto (II) [online]. 3tres3, November 2012 [accessed 2014]. Available from: http://www.3tres3.com/consejos_de_manejo/traspasos-de-lechones-hasta-3-4-dias-post-parto-ii_31654/

CASANOVAS, C. ¿Cuándo igualamos las camadas? [online] 3tres3, January 2012 [accessed 2014]. Available from: http://www.3tres3.com/consejos_de_manejo/¿cuando-igualamos-las-camadas_30503/

CASANOVAS, C. ¿Cómo igualamos las camadas tras el parto? (I) [online] 3tres3, February 2012 [accessed 2014]. Available from: http://www.3tres3.com/consejos_de_manejo/¿como-igualamos-las-camadas-tras-el-parto-i_30584/

CASANOVAS, C. ¿Cómo igualamos las camadas tras el parto? (II) Contar o no contar tetas, esa es la cuestión [online]. 3tres3, March 2012 [accessed 2014]. Available from: http://www.3tres3.com/consejos_de_manejo/¿como-igualamos-las-camadas-tras-el-parto-ii-contar-tetas_30722/

CASANOVAS, C. ¿Cómo igualamos las camadas tras el parto? (III) Igualar por número y tamaño [online]. 3tres3, July 2012 [accessed 2014]. Available from: http://www.3tres3.com/consejos_de_manejo/¿como-igualamos-las-camadas-tras-el-parto-iii-numero-y-tamaño_31253/

CASANOVAS, C. ¿Cómo igualamos las camadas tras el parto? (IV) Precauciones especiales [online]. 3tres3, August 2012 [accessed 2014]. Available from: http://www.3tres3.com/consejos_de_manejo/¿como-igualamos-las-camadas-tras-el-parto-iv-precauciones-especiales_31378/

CASANOVAS, C. Control térmico de lechones en maternidad (IV) [online]. 3tres3, March 2011 [accessed 2014]. Available from: https://www.3tres3.com/consejos_de_manejo/maternidad-control-termico-de-lechones-en-maternidad-iv_4422/

CASANOVAS, J. *Rompiendo tópicos: ¿Es el jueves el mejor día para destetar? XXXV.* Anaporc symposium. 2014.

Chiba, L.I. Section 4: Baby Pig Management (Birth to Weaning), *Swine Production Handbook*, Auburn University, 2004.

Collell, M. and Marco, E. Control ambiental en ganado porcino. Barcelona: Merial, 2008.

Collell, M. *Manejo en calor.* Sant Just Desven: Fatro Ibérica, 2009.

Collell, M. Alimentación de la cerda en gestación [online]. 3tres3, November 2007 [accessed 2014]. Available from: https://www.3tres3.com/print/1736

Collell, M. Motivación y organización del trabajo. *Suis*, 2006, 27: 64-74.

Collell, M. Gestión de recursos humanos. *Suis*, 2006, 25: 50-58.

Dourmad, J. Y. et al. La reconstitution des réserves corporelles chez la truie multipare en gestation: influence des apports d'énergie. *Journées Recherche Porcine en France*, 1991, 23:75-84.

English, P. Valoración, organización y motivación. *Suis*, 2007, 43: 55-65.

Escobet, J. *Climatización de la transición.* VETSUPPORT+ seminars for the management of the transition and fattening stages, Zaragoza, May 2013.

Evans, M. Formación para lograr el éxito. *Suis*, 2006, 25: 6-8.

Fairbrother, J. M. *Escherichia coli* en ganado porcino. *Syva Monograph*. Zaragoza: Grupo Asís, 2009.

Fernández, E. El agua de bebida: necesidades de consumo. *Avances Tecnología Porcina*, 2009, vol. VI (12): 29-30.

Fernández, E. Vitaminas en cerdas reproductoras. *Avances Tecnología Porcina*, 2009, vol. VI (5): 35-36.

Farmer, C. *The gestating and lactating sow*. Wageningen: Wageningen Academic Publishers, 2015.

Forcada, F. et al. *Ganado porcino. Diseño de alojamientos e instalaciones.* Zaragoza: Servet, 2009.

Foxcroft, G. et al. Características más importantes de las líneas maternas porcinas actuales (II). *Avances Tecnología Porcina,* 2008, vol. V (3): 4-18.

Foxcroft, G. et al. Características más importantes de las líneas maternas porcinas actuales (II). *Avances Tecnología Porcina*, 2008, vol. V (2): 4 13.

Fraile, L. *Antimicrobial therapy in swine.* Zaragoza: Servet, 2014

Frigo, E. ¿Qué es la capacitación? [online] Forodeseguridad, 2014 [accessed 2014]. Available from: http://www.forodeseguridad.com/artic/rrhh/7011.htm

Frontera, E. M. et al. *Patología parasitaria porcina.* Zaragoza: Servet, 2005.

Fruh, B. et al. *HACCP for suckling piglet mortality.* Frick: Research Institute of Organic Agriculture (FiBL), 2011.

Gadd, J. El éxito del trabajo en equipo. *Suis*, 2014, 109: 10-13.

Gadd, J. Cómo motivar a los ganaderos de porcino. *Suis*, 2014, 107: 10-13.

Gadd, J. El veterinario como instructor: buena observación. *Suis*, 2006, 25: 10-12.

Gadd, J. Cómo reconocer a un buen encargado de explotación. *Suis*, 2005, 22: 14-16

Gill, P. Colostrum: food for life [online]. The Pig Site, September 2002 [accessed 2014]. Available from: http://www.thepigsite.com/articles/677/colostrum-food-for-life

Gómez Bautista M. et al. Control de las parasitosis en porcino. *Avances Tecnología Porcina*, 2007, vol. (5): 6-22.

Gramer, D. et al. Nuevos datos sobre "viejos" patógenos: *E. coli* y Rotavirus. *Avances Tecnología Porcina*, 2010, vol. VII (9): 6-14.

Greiner, L. Alimentación de cerdas reproductoras multíparas y nulíparas. *Avances Tecnología Porcina*, 2010, vol. VII (1-2): 18-27.

Guedes, R. Avances en la detección de patógenos entéricos. *Avances Tecnología Porcina*, 2011, vol. VIII (3): 67-78.

Gyles, C.L and Fairbrother, J.M., *Escherichia coli*. In: *Pathogenesis of bacterial infections in animals* (Eds: C.L. Gyles, J.F. Prescott, J.G. Songer and C.O. Thoen), 4th ed., Oxford: Wiley-Blackwell, 2010.

Hypor. *Increasing piglet survival to weaning*, 2009.

King'ori, A. M. The pre-weaning piglet: colostrum and milk intake: a review. *Journal of Animal Production Advances*, 2012, vol. 2 (6): 277-283.

Klobasa, F. et al. Composition of sow milk during lactation. *Journal of Animal Science*, 1987, 64: 1458-1466.

Kuller, W. I. et al. Intermittent suckling: effects on piglet and sow performance before and after weaning. *Journal of Animal Science*, 2004, 82: 405-413.

Lawlor, P. How much feed do lactating sows need? [online] The Pig Site, November 2012 [accessed 2014]. Available from: http://www.thepigsite.com/articles/4143/hom-much-feed-do-lactating-sows-need

Lawlor, P., Moorepark, T. Keeping piglets in large litters alive [online]. Teagasc, November 2004 [accessed 2014]. Available from: http://www.teagasc.ie/publications/2004/20041011/paper07.asp

Le Dividich, J. *Les enjeux du colostrum.* Expo-Congrès du porc du Québec, 2006, 51-72.

Leman, A. D., Dunne, H.W. (eds.). *Diseases of swine*. Mosby, 1992.

López, M. J. *Claves para el control ambiental.* Usos en campo. Barcelona: Merial, 2007.

Lorenzo, J., Rosas, Mª. L. Mejoras en la producción de lechones en el postdestete y cerdas en lactación por el uso de acidificantes y aceites esenciales seleccionados. *Avances Tecnología Porcina*, 2008, vol. V (11): 80-84.

Mackinnon, J. D. Manejo pre-destete de los lechones: estrategias para la supervivencia, salud y crecimiento (II). *Avances Tecnología Porcina*, 2011, vol. VIII (4): 34-47.

Magallón, E. et al. *Husbandry and management practices in farrowing units I. Farrowing.* Zaragoza: Servet, 2014.

Mancera, J. C. *Controles de alimentación de la cerda hiperprolífica en lactación*, Inga Food, Zaragoza, 2010.

Manteca, X. *Etología veterinaria*. Barcelona: Multimedia Ediciones Veterinarias, 2009.

Manteca, X. et al. *Bienestar animal en el ganado porcino*. Barcelona: Boehringer, 2008.

Marco, E. Aspectos nutricionales y de manejo del pienso que influyen sobre la patología digestiva de la cerda. *Avances Tecnología Porcina*, 2009, vol. VI (3): 36-47.

Martin, C. *Datos de necesidades de las cerdas.* Nutrition and Formulation Service, Nanta S.A. 2014.

Martin, C. et al. Master 2 Know Nutreco, 2012.

Martineau, G. P., Morvan, H. and Waret-Szkuta, A. Epidermitis exudativa y necrobacilosis facial. *Suis*, 2011, 80: 44-50.

Martineau, G. P. and Badouard, B. *Managing highly prolific sows.* London Swine Conference, 2009.

Martineau, G. P. *Maladies d'élevage des porcs.* Paris: Editions France Agricole. 1997.

Mavromichalis, I. Cómo aumentar el consumo de pienso en las cerdas lactantes. *Suis*, 2013, 98: 6-8.

Mavromichalis, I. Cuestiones críticas sobre el pienso para lechones. *Suis*, 2013, 95: 6-8.

Mavromichalis, I. La importancia de la alimentación en la lactación. *Suis*, 2012, 93: 6-8.

Mavromichalis, I. Sobre posibles alternativas al uso de lactosa en lechones. *Suis*, 2004, 4: 8-10.

McCutcheon, G. Controlling energy costs [online]. Teagasc, August 2011 [accessed 2014]. Available from: http://www.teagasc.ie/publications/2011/1406/PigNewsletterAug2011.pdf.

McFarlane, J. Temperatura efectiva del entorno y confort. *Suis*, 2004, 12: 28-34.

Morillo, A. et al. La composición de las dietas de las cerdas lactantes y la producción láctea (I). *Avances Tecnologia Porcina*, 2014, vol. XI (7-8): 32-42.

Morillo, A. et al. La composición de las dietas de las cerdas lactantes y la producción láctea (I). *Avances Tecnología Porcina*, 2014, vol. XI (9): 26-44.

Muirhead, M. R., Alexander, T. *Managing Pig Health and the Treatment of Disease.* Sheffield: 5M Publishing, 1997.

Neumann, E. J. et al. *Swine disease manual*, 4th edition. USA: A.A.S.V., 2009.

Noguera, J. L. et al. Banco de datos de referencia del porcino español. *Boletín e-BDporc,* IRTA, 2014.

Oliva, J. E. *Eficiencia en maternidad*. Fatro seminar, 2014.

Palomo, A. Diarrea epidémica porcina. *Avances Tecnología Porcina*, 2013, vol. X (6): 38-39.

Palomo, A. Vitalidad de los lechones en cerdas hiperprolíficas. *Avances Tecnología Porcina*, 2011, vol. VIII (3): 50-60.

Palomo, A. XI Simposium internacional sobre fisiología digestiva en cerdos. *Avances Tecnología Porcina*, 2009, vol. VI (11): 615.

Palomo, A. Puntos clave en la patología de la nutrición porcina. *Avances Tecnología Porcina*, 2009, vol. VI (5): 38-44.

Palomo, A. Estrategias nutricionales para mejorar la salud digestiva en porcino. *Avances Tecnología Porcina*, 2009, vol. VI (4): 22-32.

Palomo, A. Gestión del personal en granjas porcinas. *Avances Tecnología Porcina*, 2008, vol. V (6): 46-51.

Palomo, A. Consumo voluntario de alimento en reproductoras. *Avances Tecnología Porcina*, 2007, vol. IV (11): 58-65.

Palomo, A. Vitalidad de los lechones en cerdas hiperprolíficas. *Avances Tecnología Porcina*, 2007, vol. IV (10): 20-34.

Palomo, A. El calostro como primer alimento del lechón. *Avances Tecnología Porcina*, 2007, vol. IV (7-8): 27-32.

Palomo, A. Alimentación líquida aplicada en ganado porcino. *Avances Tecnología Porcina*, 2006, vol. III (11): 36-40.

Palomo, A. Anemia ferropénica en lechones lactantes. *Avances Tecnología Porcina*, 2005, vol. II (4): 99-103.

Palomo, A. Necesidades vitamínicas en ganado porcino. *Avances Tecnología Porcina*, 2005, vol. II (3): 92-101.

Palomo, A. Ganancia Media Diaria en porcino. *Avances Tecnología Porcina*, 2004, vol. I (6): 74-78.

Palomo, A. Mortalidad en lechones lactantes. *Avances Tecnología Porcina*, 2004, vol. I (10): 45-57.

Pérez, J. F., Nofrarías, M. *Influencia de la nutrición sobre la patología digestiva del lechón (I).* 24th FEDNA specialisation course, 2009, vol. VI (9): 20-38.

Pinilla, J. C., Williams, A. M. Manejo de granja de hembras para alto rendimiento (II). *Avances Tecnología Porcina*, 2011, vol. VIII (1-2): 21-30.

PINILLA, J. C. et al. Strategies to reduce preweaning mortality. [en línea]. Pic.com, 2011 [accessed 2014]. Available from: http://www.pic.com/Images/Users/1/salesportal/presentations/2011BootCamp/3_Pinilla_TIPStoreduceP-WM-TSpresentationroadshow_PRINT.pdf

PLUSKE J. R. et al. *Weaning the pig: concepts and consequences.* Wageningen: Wageningen Academic Publishers, 2003.

PROBST MILLER, S. Gestión de riesgos en la sala de partos. *Suis*, 2008, 46: 40-48.

QUESNEL, H. Calostro: papel en el rendimiento del lechón y producción de la cerda. *Avances Tecnología Porcina*, 2013, vol. X (6): 14-26.

QUILES, A., ALFONSO DE VEGA, F. Principales parasitosis en el cerdo blanco: coccidiosis, helmintosis intestinales y sarna (I). *Avances Tecnología Porcina*, 2009, vol. VI (5): 20-34.

QUILES A., HEVIA M. L. *Cría y manejo del lechón.* Madrid: Acalanthis, 2006.

QUILES A., HEVIA M. L. *Manejo y alimentación de la cerda*. Madrid: Acalanthis, 2007.

QUILES A., HEVIA M. L. *Producción porcina intensiva*. Madrid: Editorial Agrícola Española, 2004.

QUINIOU, N. Condición corporal de las cerdas en maternidad. *Albéitar,* 2014, 181: 44-45.

QUINIOU, N. Nutrición de las cerdas de alto potencial. *Suis*, 2013, 96: 14-21.

QUINIOU, N. et al. Aporte suplementario de alimento o de lípidos durante los últimos 10 días de gestación y sus consecuencias sobre el parto y la lactación. *Avances Tecnología Porcina*, 2008, vol. V (11): 38-55.

REAMS, R. Y., HARRINGTON, D. D., GLICKMAN, L. T., THACKER, H. L. AND BOWERSTOCK, T. L. Multiple serotypes and strains of Streptococcus suis in naturally infected swine herds. *J. Vet. Diagn. Invest.*, 1996, 8:119-121.

REESE, D. et al. Baby pig management (Birth to weaning) [online]. eXtension, April 2010 [accessed 2014]. Available from: http://www.extension.org/pages/27050/baby-pig-management-birth-to-weaning

REINA, D. et al. Coccidiosis en porcino. *Avances Tecnología Porcina*, 2011, vol. VIII (10): 15-24.

REMAEKERS, R. *Nutrición de cerdas.* Zaragoza: Nanta, 2010.

REMAEKERS, P. *Sow feed formulation and feeding programs*. Zaragoza: Nutreco Swine Academy, 2013.

REVUELTA, M., GUILLOU, D. El periparto: el gran reto de la cerda y de su microflora intestinal. *Avances Tecnología Porcina*, 2013, vol. X (11): 26-34.

RIX, M., KETCHEM, R. Focus on farrowing to save more pigs [on line]. National Hog Farmer, 2010 [accessed 2014]. Available from: http://nationalhogfarmer.com/weekly-preview1011-focus-farrowing-save-pigs

RODRÍGUEZ, V. et al. Ventajas, inconvenientes y peculiaridades de la alimentación líquida en porcino. *Avances Tecnología Porcina*, 2010, vol. VII (9): 28-43.

RUTTEN-RAMOS, S. Optimizar la producción porcina. *Suis*, 2008, 46: 30-38.

SALÓ, N. *La comunicación en la empresa.* Barcelona: Paidós, 2005.

SANJOAQUIN, L. *Manejo de la cerda hiperprolífica.* Zaragoza: Servet, 2014.

SCHWARTZ, K. J. *Swine Disease Manual*. Iowa: American Association of Swine Veterinarians, 2004.

STALLJOHANN, G., SCHULTE-SUTRUM, R. Yoghurt for stronger suckling piglets and sows [online]. Pigprogress, April 2014 [accessed 2014]. Available from: http://www.pigprogress.net/Special-Focus/Piglet-Feeding/Yoghurt-for-stronger-suckling-piglets-and-sows/

STRAW, B. et al. *Diseases of Swine*. 8th edition. Ames, IW: Iowa State University Press, 1999.

THORUP, F. Improving piglet survival in large litters [online]. Porkcrc, 2014 [accessed 2014]. Available from: http://.porkcrc.com.au/Flemming_Thorup.ppt

VAN DEN BRAND, H. ¿Son las dietas ricas en grasa beneficiosas para las hembras lactantes? *Suis*, 2006, 28: 24-32.

VAN ENGEN, M. et al. *Pig signals: Piglets.* Best: Rooedbont. 2011.

VENTURA, J. Formación. *Suis*, 2006, 26: 52-63.

VELARDE, A., MANTECA, X. Los expertos opinan: castración quirúrgica sin anestesia [online]. 3tres3, July 2009 [accessed 2014]. Available from: http://www.3tres3.com/los-expertos-opinan/castracion-quirurgica-sin-anestesia 2652

VIGNOLA, M. *Sow feeding management during lactation.* London Swine Conference, 2009.

VILLALBA, R. et al. Producción láctea de la cerda: mayor peso, mayores crecimientos de la camada y lechones más uniformes al destete. Prueba con varios AINEs. *Avances Tecnología Porcina*, 2001, vol. I (5): 4-31.

WHITTEMORE, C. T. *The science and practice of pig production.* Arlington: Harlow Scientific and Technical Editions, 1993.

WHITTEMORE, C. T., ELSLEY F. W. H. *Practical pig nutrition*. New York: Diamond Farm Book Publishers, 1976.

ZIMMERMAN, J. J. et al. *Diseases of swine.* 10th edition. Hoboken: Wiley-Blackwell, 2012.